Quiet Thoughts, Calm Mind, the Natural Way

Traditional Simple Practices such as Abdominal Breathing, Mindfulness and Meditation to Quiet Thoughts for a Calm, Peaceful Mind

Mercedes Lemstra

BALBOA.
PRESS

A DIVISION OF HAY HOUSE

Balboa Press books may be ordered through
booksellers or by contacting:

Balboa Press
A Division of Hay House
1663 Liberty Drive
Bloomington, IN 47403
www.balboapress.com
1 (877) 407-4847

Print information available on the last page.

ISBN: 978-1-9822-0752-6 (sc)
ISBN: 978-1-9822-0751-9 (e)

Balboa Press rev. date: 07/17/2018

Acknowledgments

I WOULD LIKE to express my deepest gratitude to the many people who supported me throughout the writing of this book. While writing a book at first appears to be an individual project, soon you learn that it really does take an entire team from start to finish. To all my family and friends who listened, read, and offered suggestions, please know that you are greatly appreciated.

A heartfelt *thank you* goes to Dr. Carolyn Dean and Dr. Norman Shealy for supporting my vision of this book and allowing me to quote their remarks. Their devotion to wellness has been an inspiration to me as I achieved my own quiet thoughts and calmed my mind.

A special thanks to my friend and mentor, Faye, who was always there to encourage me and support my endeavors. When I got tongue-tied and couldn't find the right words, Faye undid the knot and got me writing again. I couldn't have done it without you!

To my good friends Correne, Nancy, Peggy, and Wanda, who so graciously agreed to try out the steps of the various exercises. Thanks, girls! Your help is greatly appreciated.

What Experts and Readers Are Saying
About
Quiet Thoughts, Calm Mind,
The Natural Way

People in the know don't tell you to take a few deep breaths for no reason! There is science behind EFT, breath work, meditation, and all the techniques that Mercedes Lemstra describes in her heartfelt book. However, the best study is when you experiment with yourself.

If there are one hundred people in a study, the number is referred to as $n=100$, but your study will be $n=1$ and every bit as valid. Take stock of your condition before you begin experimenting with the suggestions given here. List all your symptoms and feelings and concerns and put a number on a scale of one to ten as to their severity, and then put that aside. Experiment for a few weeks, then go back to your list, and see how much you have shifted by using simple methods to calm your physical, mental, and emotional body. You will be amazed, just like the investigators who take the time, money, and effort to do this research with large groups in a formal setting.

Most books that deal with stress reduction focus on one technique. However, *Quiet Thoughts, Calm Mind, The Natural Way* is a powerful book that covers six techniques, allowing you to choose the one that suits you best or to use a bit of all of them. Grab hold of this book and use it wisely to take responsibility for your own health.

Carolyn Dean, MD, ND, Creator of The Total Body ReSet—www.RnAReSet.com

Sir William Osler, the father of modern medicine, wrote extensively about stress as the cause of disease. Two reactions to stress, anxiety and depression, are the major causes of all disease, from hypertension to heart disease and cancer. Moreover, these dominant emotional disturbances contribute to the rampant disease epidemic we now observe.

The antidote to all of these problems is practical relaxation as discussed in the book by Mercedes Lemstra, *Quiet Thoughts, Calm Mind, The Natural Way*. With detailed attention to breathing, mindfulness, gratitude, Autogenic Training, Meditation and Emotional Freedom Technique, you have here the answer to health of body, mind, and emotions. With all six practices in one book, try them all out to find the ones that best quiet your thoughts, calm your mind, and relax your body.

C. Norman Shealy, MD, PhD

Founder and CEO, International Institute of Holistic Medicine

Mercedes Lemstra has become my "health guru" for all natural means of maintaining a healthy body and mind. Having known Mercedes throughout the time she conducted her own search for the ultimate quiet mind, I have witnessed the maze of personal and professional experiences and research she went through, culminating in the writing of this wonderful book so that others may benefit.

Speaking for myself as someone who always had a constantly active mind, previously uninformed about specific solutions like these for achieving calmness of mind, the detailed descriptions of activities and steps in *Quiet Thoughts, Calm Mind, The Natural Way* have made the calming process easy to understand, envision, and finally transfer to action. For anyone who is just beginning his or her own study and practice, the tried-and-true suggestions in this book may be the perfect start of your own calm mind.

Faye Crow, author and publisher of *Ready Reading, a Multisensory Approach to Beginning Reading*—www. readyreading.com

Quiet Thoughts, Calm Mind, The Natural Way is the perfect book to get anyone started on calming his or her anxious mind. There is just enough information to understand how the mind works without it becoming overwhelming. The step-by-step approach makes doing the exercises simple and easy. For anyone trying to calm their mind in a natural way without drugs, this is certainly the book to help you do that. Moreover, the six most popular ways to calm the mind are all included in this one book.

Chris L., a reader

This book is the ideal place to start for anyone trying to quiet his or her thoughts in a natural way. The individual exercises within the six practices are clearly explained in an easy-to-follow way. All the tips and suggestions clear away any confusion about the best way to do the exercises. I highly recommend *Quiet Thoughts, Calm Mind, The Natural Way* to anyone interested in calming their mind in a more natural holistic way.

Viola C., a reader

CONTENTS

INTRODUCTION

IN THIS BOOK, you will find tried-and-true, simple, and easy natural practices that bring peace of mind by quieting your thoughts. It is not intended to be an in-depth study of any of the practices. Rather, it is meant to be an introduction to these simple but highly effective practices that have been used, individually or in combination, for centuries to effectively quiet thoughts, calm the mind, and relax the body.

You won't find any lengthy research studies or charts. Nor will you find graphs of the results of meta-analyses. There will be a minimum of expert quotes or long-winded scientific explanations. Where scientific research supports the benefits of the practice, I have included the results of that research.

I have also included the possible benefits that you may experience as you practice these exercises because I feel it's important for you to know why anyone would want to practice them in the first place. Knowing what the benefits are may also help you decide on one exercise over another, depending on your special situation or circumstance.

Each section can be read independently and the exercises done without reading the other sections, with one exception. In the first section, Breathwork, diaphragmatic breathing, or abdominal breathing is explained. This breathing exercise can be incorporated as part of any or all of the other exercises once you become familiar and comfortable doing it.

For this reason, I highly recommend that if you skip Part One, you begin by reading the Breathwork section in Part Two to familiarize yourself with abdominal breathing. This is the first breathing exercise detailed in that section. Practice this breathing exercise until you feel comfortable with it and can do it easily. You can then use it as a stand-alone exercise to calm your mind or together with any of the other exercises.

In Part One, I've given relevant information about what stress is and how the body responds to stressors. I've gone into more detail because I feel that it is important to understand how and why the body responds in the way it does. Knowing how the body responds to stress makes it easy to understand why you are experiencing the specific sensations, reactions, emotions, and feelings. I've tried to be thorough without getting too medical or technical.

Throughout Part Two, I may repeat an explanation that I've already covered in Part One in greater detail.

This ensures that if readers skipped Part One, they will still have enough information to understand what is causing the feelings and reactions they are experiencing.

One other important consideration is that this book is not intended in any way, shape, or form to be taken as medical advice. If you are having questionable symptoms that concern you, please make an appointment to discuss this with your medical adviser. This enables you to make a wise decision on the best approach to address your specific individual concern, which may include these natural practices.

I am not a medical doctor, nor am I a naturopath, nor do I play one on TV! My intention is not to offer these practices as medical advice in any way. These practices are included because after much research and trial and error on my part, I have found them to work well in quieting my runaway mind.

In this busy day and age, I wish I'd had a book like this to get me started with some easy-to-implement, practical exercises during my times of racing thoughts and stressful moments. Instead, I learned of these one by one after much research, which took a lot of time and effort. It is my sincere hope that you, the reader, will be spared all that research and hours of reading to say nothing of the expense.

If at any time you're unsure of the meaning of a term or are just intrigued by a concept and want more information, don't hesitate to do an Internet search.

You will find countless websites and much information to help clarify the concept. For example, if you are unfamiliar with who Darth Vader was or have no idea how his breathing sounded, a search on the Internet will offer many pages filled with sites to visit to learn more. I have included resources at the back of this book to get you started.

For the most part, by practicing these simple and yet very effective exercises, your mind may begin to find some peace and tranquility. Regardless of why your mind is running away with itself, whether your worries are financial, relationships, family, or any of the other many issues we choose to worry about, these practices may guide you on the road to quieting your thoughts and calming your runaway mind.

In order for these practices to be effective, one suggestion is to begin practicing them at a time when your mind isn't in the middle of a runaway crisis. Begin by practicing the exercise several times, ideally every day, several times a day during the times when your mind is calm. Once your mind has experienced this calm, it will associate the calm and relaxed feeling with the exercise, using it as a reference point and returning to it easily.

This pattern of calmness is established with repeated practice on a regular basis. As the mind settles into the familiar practice that produces calmness, it quiets those racing thoughts while relaxing the body. It makes it much easier to quickly and easily fall into the rhythm of peaceful breathing, quietude, and relaxation. This is the key to the success of these practices.

As we begin our journey into relieving stress and calming our mind the natural way, let's spend a little time understanding exactly what stress is and how the body responds to and handles stress. Taking the time to understand the connection between the mind and body will bring a new wisdom to how quieting the thoughts can change many aspects in your life for the better. Once the mind is calm, after using the exercises included with each practice, we can easily see how the body follows suite and relaxes.

PART ONE

ALL ABOUT STRESS

STRESSED DEFINED

STRESS IS A factor in everyday life for all of us. It is often described as a feeling of being overwhelmed, feeling tired but wired, sleepy and yet unable to sleep, worrying, and feeling tense all the time. It has become a buzzword we hear everywhere. However, most of us are too stressed to find the time to try to understand the stress response that we are experiencing or to research ways to relieve it.

As we watch the daily news, we see images that cause us to feel sad, angry, stressed, or horrified. Sometimes we carry these images in our mind throughout our day, causing us to feel that same stress over and over again. We may even discuss what we've seen while at work, which keeps the stress alive and anchored in our mind and body.

Perhaps the situation that you are experiencing is with someone in your life. Feelings of anger and resentment stay with you day in and day out, causing you to feel hopeless or discouraged. You feel like you have nowhere to turn and live with that constant stress in your body on a daily basis. This unresolved chronic stress has a very toxic effect on your body.

Everyone responds to stress in a different way. This may offer a snapshot into how and why we feel what we feel, how we process our experiences, and how healthy we are. As we explore the fascinating subject of stress, we may get some insight into why it is so important to respond to stress in a way that is not harmful to the body.

It is important to know that everyone feels stressed at one time or another. Some people respond and cope with stress more effectively than others. Some people recover from stressful situations more quickly than others do. It is important to develop an awareness of how you respond to stress, whether minor or major, chronic or acute, in order to understand how it is affecting you.

WHAT IS STRESS?

The heading to this section is a bit of a misnomer because stress is such a subjective concept that it is hard to define. Stress means different things to different people. To Hans Selye, a Hungarian endocrinologist who is credited with coining the word "stress," it meant the nonspecific response of an organism to a stressor or to a demand.

That leads us to define what a stressor is. The *Merriam-Webster* dictionary defines stressor as "a physical, chemical, or emotional factor that causes bodily or mental tension and may be a factor in disease causation." In other words, a stressor is any person, event, thing, or circumstance that places a demand on our body and upsets our emotional, mental, or physical balance.

Any type of stressor or demand, such as work, exercise, traumatic experiences, life changes, or school, places stress on the body. Since stressors appear to be everywhere, it is impossible to avoid them in our daily life. It is not the stressor that is the concern; it is how the body and the mind respond to each stressor that is important.

SIGNS OF STRESS

When the body is experiencing stress, it experiences the fight-or-flight response. The body produces the stress hormones, cortisol and adrenaline, which prepare the body for either fighting or fleeing the threat, hence the name. The body responds in this way whether the stress is perceived or real. More detail on this in the next section.

If the stress is ongoing or chronic, you may experience some common symptoms. Some of the symptoms may be physical or behavioral, while others may be emotional or mental. Since these responses are not exclusive to stress, it is important to determine what other causes could be causing the symptoms you are experiencing to rule out other illnesses.

Here are some of the more common emotional or mental symptoms that you may experience or that may intensify during times of chronic stress:

- Anxiety
- Racing thoughts
- Feeling overwhelmed, out of control
- Feeling sad, moody, teary
- Low self-esteem, lack of self-confidence
- Difficulty concentrating or focusing
- Irritability, anger
- Fatigue
- Depression

Some of the more common physical symptoms that may occur during chronic stress are these:

- Headaches, other aches and pains
- Upset stomach, indigestion, nausea
- Rapid heartbeat
- Stiff neck or tight shoulders
- Sweaty palms and generalized sweating
- Feeling tense, unable to relax
- Insomnia
- Unable to fall asleep after waking in the middle of the night
- Fast breathing
- Weight problems
- Loss of memory

Stress can also have an effect on your behavior. Here are some common ways that people react to stress:

- Excessive anger or angry outbursts
- Withdrawal from social contacts
- Alcohol abuse
- Drug abuse
- Overeating or under eating
- Insomnia or sleeping too much
- Nervous habits such as nail biting or pacing

Over time, stress may also produce specific conditions in the different organs or organ systems in the body. Here are some of the changes felt in different parts of the body:

Heart: Chronic stress may be linked to high blood pressure, arrhythmias, hardening of the arteries, blood clots, and even heart failure.

Lungs: Stress may intensify symptoms of allergies, asthma, and COPD.

Stomach: Stress can make stomach reflux (GERD), ulcers, and irritable bowel syndrome worst.

Skin: Stress can make the skin reactions such as acne and psoriasis more acute.

It is also important to note that not all stress is bad. Selye also coined the word "eustress" for stress that is good stress. For example, good stress can help you prepare for and win a race. Running and building resistance in preparation for the race is stressful for the body. However, once the race is over, the stress generally disappears and the body returns to normal.

Another example of good stress happens when you are in danger while driving and need to react quickly to a situation in order to avoid a car accident. Usually this stress lasts for a short time, and the body returns to normal quickly. This short-term stress is usually not harmful to the body. However, it is necessary to help us get through the stressful activity or situation we find ourselves in.

Eustress has some general benefits such as:

- focusing our energy
- motivating us to complete our task
- energizing us
- increasing our feeling of well-being
- increasing our performance
- increasing our feelings of accomplishment
- increasing self-confidence

TYPES OF STRESS

Generally speaking, there are four major categories of stress. I've placed the four types of stress in a grid to make it easier to understand. This way the relationship between the different types of stress can be easily seen and understood. I refer to the good stress as "eustress" to distinguish it from the undesirable stress, "distress." Let's begin by defining what each term means.

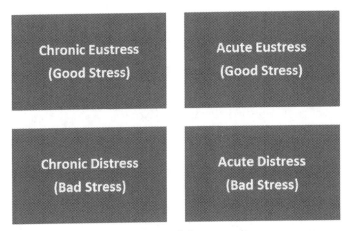

Types of Stress

CHRONIC EUSTRESS

When we refer to chronic eustress, we are talking about the very best kind of stress to have. Chronic eustress is long-lasting recurring stress of the good kind. When we are in a state of chronic eustress, all the body systems are working in harmony with each other for an optimal healthy state. The different body systems are producing the feel-good hormones like serotonin, oxytocin, and dopamine. This allows all the cells in the body to be bathed in a cocktail of well-being and feel-good hormones. The result is optimal health and a sense of complete well-being.

The feelings flooding our body while we are in this state are love, joy, peace, happiness, self-fulfillment, and contentment. We are generally very satisfied with our life and feel very self-confident. We feel like life is going our way, and we have control over what happens to us. Adding these feelings to the feel-good hormones circulating in the body creates a wonderful healthy environment for the body to complete all the processes needed for optimal health.

An example of this type of stress is a happily married couple who have many activities that they enjoy doing together. They enjoy spending time in each other's company; they have many common interests and enjoy doing things, which they both like, together. They generally feel happy and content spending time with each other. If there are disagreements, they are quickly resolved with little or no lingering resentment or anger. In general, life is good!

It is almost impossible to maintain a state of chronic eustress indefinitely. However, as we discuss all the aspects of stress, it will be easier to find ways to maintain this very desirable state often throughout the ups and downs of daily living. Once you recognize the ways in which your body responds to the different kinds of stress, you will be able to find ways to relieve the stress you are feeling and return to the optimal state of chronic eustress. The practices introduced in this book will start you on your way to relieving the stress that you encounter on a daily basis to prevent it from becoming chronic stress.

ACUTE EUSTRESS

Acute usually refers to a condition that appears rapidly, is of short duration, and usually is intense. This is exactly what acute eustress is. It is stress that has a quick onset, is intense, but doesn't last very long. This kind of eustress is good for the body to experience.

An example of acute eustress is the stress you feel when you receive particularly good news that you've been hoping for a long time. You feel that rush of all the feel-good hormones come on quickly and intensely. You are ecstatic as you share the long-awaited news with family and friends, but once the moment is finished, the body returns to its normal state.

CHRONIC DISTRESS

As the word "chronic" indicates, chronic distress is stress that is of long duration, reappears, and may cause a whole host of conditions in the body. When we are experiencing chronic stress, the body is flooded with the stress hormones, cortisol and adrenaline, which keep the body in a state of chronic fight-or-flight. This state interferes with the normal body functions needed to digest as well as assimilate food; protect the body from bacteria or other invaders; and leaves the immune system and the body in a weakened, vulnerable condition. This state is by far the most harmful for the body.

The longer the body stays in this state, the more likely you are to develop any of a host of serious illnesses such as heart arrhythmias or heart disease, diabetes, mental and emotional problems, and the list goes on. This is the state you want to get yourself out of as quickly as possible and find ways to make sure you do not return to. Sometimes the only way may be to leave the situation causing you that degree of stress, if it's possible, no matter how difficult that decision may seem. In the long run, you'll be glad you did.

Sometimes it is impossible to remove yourself from a situation causing chronic stress. An example of this would be someone experiencing chronic emphysema. People with chronic emphysema most likely have had the condition for a long time. Having this condition impacts their ability to breathe normally and also their quality of life, easily causing chronic distress in the body. Having to be responsible for the equipment needed to breathe while performing daily duties just adds to the stress of not being able to breathe easily and effortlessly.

ACUTE DISTRESS

Acute distress is bad stress that appears rapidly, is of short duration, and feels intense. Usually this stress may not feel like much fun, but it doesn't last long and is quickly forgotten. An example of this type of stress is what you would feel being in a narrow escape in a car during rush hour. It would come on quickly and very intensely as you saw the impending danger, but once you had swerved to safety, it would pass within a short time.

Our body is equipped to handle this kind of stress very efficiently. The body goes into fight-or-flight as it reacts to the impending danger, again producing the stress hormones, cortisol and adrenaline. These hormones make it possible for you to react in a quick-decisive manner to avoid the impending accident. Once the danger is over, the body breaks down the hormones, and they are removed, leaving the body in a state of harmony once again. No lingering harmful effects remain to do any damage to the body.

Even though the body can handle this kind of stress quite efficiently, and it appears to be harmless, it is not a good idea to place the body in situations of acute stress often. Any amount of bad stress, done to extremes, will take its toll on the body.

It is when stress is ongoing for longer periods of time, day after day, that the body begins to feel the harmful effects of the chronic stress. As mentioned previously our body is very capable of handling short-term distress without harmful consequences. However, it is when stress is caused by a situation that lasts for long periods and becomes chronic stress that it can have serious consequences and contribute to serious health problems.

MAJOR AREAS OF STRESS

As stated previously, chronic stress is found in all areas of our lives. Sometimes it has become a way of life so much so that we don't even realize that we are experiencing any stress at all. We assume that the way we are feeling is "just the normal way for us."

The areas listed below illustrate just how pervasive chronic stress can be in our daily personal lives. In many cases, we are not living with chronic stress in just one of these areas but in several of them at the same time. This compounds the harmful effect of chronic stress on our body.

Family relationships. Family relationships can be particularly stressful if you have children who have emotional or physical challenges. If you are caring for an elderly or ill parent, this can cause tremendous stress on the caregiver. If you feel alone or unsupported, that can cause the stress you feel to multiply exponentially.

Health. If you are dealing with a chronic illness like diabetes, heart disease, or arthritis, the stress just compounds. For those living in chronic pain, the stress is ever present 24-7. Studies have shown that the stress you feel because of your condition can even make the condition worst.

Emotional problems. Studies have shown that repressed emotions like anger or resentment place much emotional stress on the body, increasing anxiety. Other feelings that place stress on the body are shame, guilt, low self-esteem, lack of self-worth, or lack of confidence. These strong emotions can contribute to illness in the body.

Major life changes. These events are very stressful and may become chronic distress if the person isn't careful to deal with them with counseling or other means when they occur. Some examples of events in this area that may cause immense stress are divorce, catastrophic illness, losing your job, or death of a spouse, parent, or child.

Living conditions. If you are forced to live in an unsafe, undesirable, or noisy neighborhood, due to financial issues, this would place great chronic distress on the body. Feeling safe and comfortable in your home is one way to destress after a long day at work.

Work conditions. If you aren't satisfied at work, don't feel valued at your job, or found the job to be too difficult for you to perform in a satisfactory manner, this would become chronically stressful.

Now that we have a better understanding of what stress is and how pervasive it is throughout our lives, let's move on to discover how our body responds to all the stressors that are found all around us. The next section will help you understand the importance of responding to stress in a way that will not produce all those physical reactions that so many of us experience that can be so harmful to the body and our health.

SECTION 2

THE STRESS RESPONSE

MANY INDIVIDUAL ORGANS and organ systems make up the human body. When all the systems are supporting each other and working in harmony, we say that the body is in a state of homeostasis. The origin of the word "homeostasis" is from the Greek words "same" and "steady." This is the optimal state where all functions and processes in the body are completed by the different organ systems, working harmoniously, with the least amount of stress.

Some of the principal organ systems are the digestive system, the circulatory system, the endocrine system, the respiratory system, and the nervous system. We will study the nervous system in this section since this system is closely associated with the stress response.

All parts of the body are connected to the central nervous system, a complex network of cells and nerves. Its function is to transmit messages from the brain and spine to the different parts of the body. The nervous system provides nerves to organs, muscles, and all other parts of the body.

Within the central nervous system, there are various systems, but we will focus on two specific systems since they play a crucial role in the body's response to stress. These two systems are the sympathetic and the parasympathetic nervous system. They are a part of the autonomic nervous system.

I have also included a brief explanation of the vagus nerve since it is also involved in stimulating the parasympathetic nervous system and is influenced by abdominal breathing. This is so important for countering the effects of the sympathetic nervous system, but I'm getting ahead of myself.

SYMPATHETIC VERSUS PARASYMPATHETIC NERVOUS SYSTEM

Here is a brief and simplified explanation of these two parts of the autonomic nervous system. When we use the word "autonomic," it helps to think "automatic." The autonomic nervous system is responsible for countless processes in the body that go on automatically without our conscious control. Some examples are breathing, digesting, heart rate, respiration, blood pressure, body temperature, swallowing, and sneezing.

The sympathetic nervous system (SNS) and the parasympathetic nervous system (PNS) are the two systems of the autonomic nervous system that contribute to the stress response or the rest-and-digest response respectively in the body. When the body is in the state of homeostasis, these two systems act in close collaboration, balancing each other to maintain the optimal state of homeostasis in the body.

When the body is not in the state of homeostasis, these two systems act in opposition to each other. The sympathetic nervous system generally stimulates the body when it needs to protect itself from real or perceived imminent danger. It contributes to what is generally known as the fight-or-flight response.

On the other hand, the parasympathetic nervous system relaxes the body during restful-peaceful times when there is no danger. It is responsible for the rest-and-digest state, or as I like to call it, the rest-and-relax state. If the activity of the SNS is increased, as in the fight-or-flight response, there is a corresponding decrease in the activity of the PNS, the rest-and-relax state.

THE BODY'S RESPONSE TO STRESS

The fight-or-flight response, a survival mechanism, is the response of the body to a real or perceived danger or threat. In the past, this response ensured our survival during times of imminent danger. However, as times changed the fight-or-flight response, that was intended to keep us safe, is now sabotaging our own bodies and minds.

In the times of our hunter-gatherer ancestors, most threats encountered were real. For example, they could be out hunting and see several tigers. The tigers represented real danger requiring them to make a decision. They could either stay and fight the tigers or take flight by running away. They had to decide quickly which of the two choices to take. There was no time to debate the pros and cons of either decision.

When you perceive a threat, the amygdala, which is the alert system in the body, sends out the danger signal. The amygdala is also the storehouse for memories. If the perceived danger matches a memory stored in the amygdala, the amygdala "hijacks" the front part of the "thinking brain," the neocortex. The result is that you are not able to think logically but go into the automatic fight-or-flight response.

This response is meant to give you a quick way of removing yourself safely from any real or perceived threat without having to think it through. The amygdala is able to process this information milliseconds faster than the thinking brain can. Since the amygdala has "hijacked" the neocortex making it impossible to think logically, the emotional response may be exaggerated or irrational. Nevertheless, the fight-or-flight response automatically kicks in.

Signals also go to the adrenal glands to prepare the body to either fight the danger or flee to get away. The adrenals respond by producing the stress hormones cortisol and adrenaline. These two hormones prepare the body to carry out successfully either choice, running away or staying to fight. This explains the name fight-or-flight given to this response state.

Two important components of the fight-or-flight response that we are focusing on here are the amygdala and the adrenal glands. The adrenal glands sit like tiny pyramids atop the kidneys, one on each kidney. They are responsible, as stated previously, for producing the hormones cortisol and adrenaline. The two hormones are important in regulating the fight-or-flight response. Hormones are chemical messengers that help regulate different body functions.

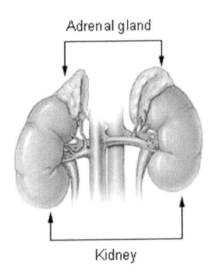

Adrenal gland

Kidney

The other key component of this fear-filled state is the amygdala, a small pea-size, almond-shaped gland. Although there are two of them, one on each side of the brain, they are usually referred to in the singular. The amygdala is located deep in the brain as can be seen in the graphic. It is important because as part of the limbic system of the brain, it is greatly involved in alerting the body to danger resulting in the fight-or-flight response.

It is also involved in processing emotions such as fear, anger, and pleasure. The effects of the amygdala can also be seen when a person reacts with explosive laughter after hearing a funny joke. Intense moments of joy also are the result of the influence of the amygdala.

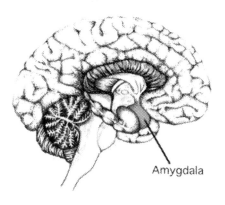

Amygdala

Today we don't encounter tigers or bears that require us to fight them or flee from them. However, the amygdala triggers the same response, the fight-or-flight response, when we face an angry boss, financial difficulties, too little sleep, or chronic stress. The amygdala senses danger whether real or perceived. This threat of danger causes the amygdala to stimulate the glands and the sympathetic nervous system to action. The adrenal glands then produce the hormones cortisol and adrenaline that cause the changes in the body in preparation to fight or flee the danger.

As you can see from this list, the changes in the body in response to the fight-or-flight state caused by the release of the hormones cortisol and adrenaline are all about preparing the body to defend itself from danger whether perceived or real. The major changes are:

- Increased heart rate for better circulation
- Elevated blood pressure for greater blood flow
- Increased blood flow to the extremities
- Widened pupils to allow for better sight
- Faster, more shallow breathing
- Shut down of the immune system
- Decreased blood flow to the digestive system
- Decreased digestion
- A general sense of impending danger

Other changes may take place in the body when it is under the effects of the fight-or-flight response. These are more subtle changes that may not be as apparent or as noticeable as the ones mentioned above. Here are some examples.

- It may interfere with learning.
- It may lower bone density.
- It may increase cholesterol.
- It may lower our resiliency to deal with daily life.
- It may interfere with our memory.
- It may cause an increase in weight gain.
- It may interfere with decision-making

In today's times, even though most of the threats we experience are not tigers or bears coming to attack us, we still experience the fight-or-flight response.

Since the amygdala does not recognize the difference between the threat of the bear and the threat of our feeling overwhelmed or afraid, it still sounds the alert.

When we have a long list of to-dos and feel anxious about accomplishing all the items on that list, and add to that accomplishing them perfectly, the amygdala reacts with the fight-or-flight response. We feel our heart beat faster; we become anxious and short-tempered; we feel overwhelmed; we have difficulty making a decision; and we can't seem to think straight. This is one reason why psychologists often recommend that you should not make important decisions if you are under severe distress.

THE PARASYMPATHETIC NERVOUS SYSTEM

The opposing nervous system to the SNS is the parasympathetic nervous system (PNS). It has the opposite effect on the body. It prepares the body for rest and relaxation as can be seen in the following list. The PNS is responsible for the relaxation response in the body characterized by:

- Normal, regular heart rate
- Decreased blood pressure
- Normal blood flow to the extremities
- Increased blood flow to the core
- More relaxed, deeper breathing
- Normal activity of the immune system
- Normal digestion and assimilation

- A sense of peace and calm
- Pupils return to their normal size

VAGUS NERVE

The vagus nerve also plays a key role in managing the effects of the parasympathetic nervous system throughout the body. The word "vagus" comes from the Latin, which means wanderer. This represents exactly how this nerve wanders throughout the body producing its calming and relaxing effects through various organs to include the heart, lungs, and stomach.

The amount of activity of the vagus nerve or its "vagal tone" determines its influence on the PNS in the body. The greater the vagal tone the faster your body can relax after a stressful event. In other words, the more active the vagus nerve is, the faster you will feel relaxed and calm resulting in greater mental and physical well-being.

Studies have found that one of the best ways to stimulate your vagus nerve is by slow, deep breathing such as abdominal breathing, which is detailed in the next section. By breathing slowly and deeply, you activate the vagus nerve that helps stimulate the PNS. The result is a calmer mind with less anxiety and a more relaxed body.

Most people take about ten to fourteen breaths per minute. Slowing your breath down to six breaths per minute is a great way to stimulate the vagus nerve and reduce anxiety. The breaths should be the abdominal breaths that allow the abdomen to expand on the inhale and contract toward the spine on the exhale. This type of breathing is key to stimulating the vagus nerve. This breathing exercise will be explained in more detail in the Breathwork section to follow.

When we are tense and anxious, in a fight-or-flight state, the activity of the SNS is most noticeable at the expense of the calming effect of the PNS and the tone of the vagus nerve. The reason for wanting to balance the activity of the SNS and the PNS, and to increase vagal tone, is to return the body to homeostasis, the optimal state of harmony and well-being within the body.

When these two nervous systems along with their cohort, the vagus nerve, are working in harmony, there is a general sense of physical and emotional well-being. The body is flooded with the good hormones serotonin and oxytocin, and a general feeling of wellness and calm pervades all the cells of the body. This allows all the organ systems, while bathed in this wellness cocktail, to perform all the necessary functions needed in order to maintain optimal health in the body easily and efficiently.

Now that we have a better understanding of what stress is, how it affects the body, and how the body responds to stress, we can begin learning the different practices that will help us quiet our thoughts to calm the mind and relax the body.

PART TWO

PRACTICES TO CALM THE MIND

General Suggestions
Section 1: Breathwork
Section 2: Mindfulness
Section 3: Gratitude
Section 4: Autogenic Training or
Autogenic Relaxation
Section 5: Meditation
Section 6: Emotional Freedom Technique (EFT)

General Suggestions

Before we get started on learning the exercises within the individual practices, I have included a list of general suggestions that apply to most of the exercises. In some instances, if there is a suggestion that is particularly important for the success of one of the exercises, I've repeated it briefly before giving the sequence for that exercise.

Morning, Evening, or In-Between

There really isn't a best time of the day to introduce or practice any of these exercises in your daily life with the exception of meditation. More details on this are given later in the Meditation section. One truly important thing is to find a time when you will not be disturbed for at least ten to thirty minutes, depending on the exercise you are practicing. At some point, you may find that ten to thirty minutes just is not enough time. You'll love the calmness that you feel and will want to remain in that calm state for a longer time. And that is perfectly fine!

BE COMFORTABLE

It's important that for all these exercises, you sit where *you* are most comfortable. If you choose to sit on the floor cross-legged, placing a pillow under your "sit" bones might be more comfortable. More on the sit bones later on.

Others find that sitting directly on the floor without the use of pillows feels just fine. This is a purely personal choice. Experiment with different ways to find the one that works best for you. Remember, this is all about *you*.

If you choose to sit in a chair, that will work just fine too as long as it is a comfortable position for you. You can sit cross-legged in the chair if you'd like. Or you can place your feet flat on the floor. If it feels comfortable, take your shoes off and place your bare feet in contact with the floor. This helps your body ground itself.

AMBIANCE...ABSOLUTELY!

There are many ways to add a relaxing, nurturing, healing ambiance while practicing these exercises. The first way that comes to mind is by adding soothing, relaxing, background music. Listening to soft gentle

Zen music helps to calm the mind as well as relax the body.

Even if you don't especially like classical music, give Baroque music for relaxation a try. It seems to soothe the mind by quiet thoughts quite easily and quickly. If you already have your favorite relaxing music, then by all means, listen to that as you relax during your practice!

Adding candles is another way to add a relaxing feeling and fragrance to the practice. You can try one of the traditional relaxing fragrances such as lavender, vanilla, or jasmine. It's also easy to find candles that combine scents such as vanilla and lavender in one candle. One other combination that is particularly effective and quite popular for relieving stress and relaxing the body is lavender with tangerine. Any of these will work provided you like the scent.

Essential oils have become very popular of late. They have a calming effect on the limbic system of the brain that includes the amygdala. This is the little almond-shaped gland responsible for the fight-or-flight response in the body. It's the body's very own alarm system! The amygdala is active when we are under stress that makes us feel anxious and afraid.

Using essential oils reduces the fearful feelings that accompany this stress response. To calm the feelings of anxiety, lavender, rosemary, patchouli, and sandalwood are very effective. One way to enjoy these essential oils is to use a diffuser. To the water in the diffuser, add a few drops of your favorite scent. It is also very effective to mix a few drops of several of your favorite oils. Experiment with this to find the most pleasing combination for you.

There are also many premixed essential oil combinations prepared especially for reducing anxiety and stress. These premixed combinations may include two or more complementary scents that together have a synergistic effect on calming the mind. While it's fun to experiment on your own, it might be easier to start by trying one of the already mixed combinations.

Essential oils can also be used very effectively by rubbing them gently on the wrist, soles of the feet, or temples. Before using essential oils directly on the skin, dilute them in a drop or two of a carrier oil. Some recommended carrier oils are sweet-almond oil, jojoba oil, sesame oil, and coconut oil. A word of caution: essential oils are a powerful gift from nature and can sometimes irritate the skin if used without diluting in a carrier oil first.

Again, try diluting the essential oil and carrier oil in equal parts first. If you find that the mixture irritates your skin, then add a few more drops of the carrier oil. On the other hand, if you find that the mixture doesn't irritate your skin, you can always add more of the essential oil, one drop at a time, to increase the concentration and fragrance.

Using a carrier oil does not dilute the effect of the essential oil. After diluting the essential oil in the carrier oil of your choice, put a little dab on your skin to see if there is any reaction. You may feel a very hot sensation, a "burning" sensation, or a prickly feel when you apply the oil. Continue diluting the essential oil until you feel no sensation on the skin when the diluted oil is applied.

When using essential oils on the skin, you can also blend two or more to create your own mix. Experiment with this until you find the perfect blend for you. One or two drops of lavender oil mixed with vanilla in a carrier oil of your choice can be very relaxing when rubbed on the temple or soles of the feet. This is a fun way to treat yourself to a relaxing experience.

TO SIT OR STAND OR LIE DOWN

As mentioned above, whether you practice sitting in a chair or on the floor is entirely up to you. Here are a few things to remember:

- ➤ When sitting in a chair or on the floor, hold your back straight—not in a tense manner, but rather in a relaxed, soft way.
- ➤ Lower your shoulders away from your ears.
- ➤ Try not to lean against the back of the chair.
- ➤ Adding a pillow behind your back may give added support.
- ➤ Sitting cross-legged on a chair is also fine; remember to keep your spine straight.

At some point, you may find yourself stressing, your mind racing out of control, some place that is not home. If you are out-and-about, standing in line at the bank or grocery store, or anywhere it is impractical to sit, it's perfectly fine to practice standing up. Once you have practiced these exercises for a while, you'll find your favorite exercise that works best for you to relieve the stress you are feeling when you are away from home. You can always do a few abdominal breathing rounds as explained in the next section.

Another breathing exercise that works well when you are away from home is the 4-7-8 Breathing exercise. As you focus your mind on keeping count, this becomes a way to quiet your thoughts because it's almost impossible to have racing thoughts and count at the same time. During this exercise, you are fully aware of what is going on around you, but at the same time, the counting is helping the mind become calm.

While lying down might sound and feel appealing, lying down is sure to relax you enough that you may fall asleep, especially if you are not getting enough rest throughout the night. While it's good that you get some rest, it doesn't help you practice the exercise. For this reason, at the beginning of your practice, I suggest that you do the exercises sitting comfortably rather than lying down.

Loose Is Best

It's best to wear loose-fitting clothes that do not restrict your breathing in any way since you can practice abdominal breathing with all the exercises. I'll explain more on abdominal breathing later.

I like to wear bottoms that have an elastic waist, which allow for the unrestricted expansion of the abdomen on the inhalation. This gives the feeling of freedom, a very relaxing and calming feeling all its own.

Straight Spine

As mentioned above, be sure to sit, whether on the floor or in a chair, with a straight spine. Also, make every effort to sit on your sit or sits bones, which helps to keep your spine straight.

You may be wondering where in the world these "sit bones" with the funny name are. When you sit straight, you are sitting on your sit bones. You literally balance yourself on these when you sit up straight. The reason we may not be aware of them is that most of us usually have a bit of padding there, which makes it difficult to feel them!

When your back is straight, it allows for easy, unrestricted flow of the air into the lungs because the abdomen can expand and contract with ease. Sitting on your sit bones allows for this in a very natural way. More details on this in the section on abdominal breathing.

To Close or Not to Close...Your Eyes

Whether to close your eyes or not depends on the exercise. If you are practicing breathing exercises, it's a matter of what feels most comfortable to you. I prefer to close mine to block out any visual distractions that might keep my focus on something other than the movement of my abdomen with each inhalation and exhalation.

It's easier for me to get into the rhythm of deep, calm breathing when my dominant awareness is of the breath moving through my body and not on what I am seeing in the room. Without any of the visual stimuli to distract me, I can easily enter into a very relaxed state because my awareness is primarily on my breathing.

For mindfulness, you can have it both ways, depending on the mindfulness exercise you are practicing. If you are practicing mindfulness while cleaning, eating, or getting dressed in the morning before work, then you most definitely want to have your eyes open. However, if you are practicing a mindful breathing exercise, then it would be perfectly fine to close your eyes.

When meditating, it's best to close the eyes. It is much easier, again, to focus on releasing your thoughts if you don't have any visual distractions. Most of our minds don't need any help in being distracted, which looking around the room during Meditation would surely do!

START QUIETLY

When you first begin any of the exercises, whichever one you are doing, allow yourself time to sit quietly for a few minutes while breathing naturally. It's amazing how quickly your mind and body learn to respond to this quiet time by becoming more relaxed. Your thoughts will begin to slow down, you'll feel your body relax with each exhalation, and your mind will feel calmer just by sitting quietly for a few minutes, breathing slowly and deeply, before actually beginning the exercise.

At this time, just breathe naturally. Don't try to control your breath. Just let the air enter through your nose in a natural way and then exhale through the nose again without controlling the rate. If it feels natural to pause after each inhalation and exhalation, do so. However, if you have to force this, just wait for a later time when you are more comfortable with the exercise and are able to pause without feeling stressed.

INCREASING MINDFULNESS

When you sit breathing quietly and focusing on your breath before beginning any exercise, you are increasing mindfulness in a very natural way. Your focus is on each breath. Think about each inhalation with each in-breath. Feel the breath enter through your nostrils. Become aware of whether your breath feels cool or warm. Listen to your breath to hear if it is quiet or raspy, steady or choppy, fast or slow, deep or shallow. Maybe you don't have any awareness of how it feels or sounds. That's OK too. But continue to focus on the breath, becoming more aware of each breath.

As you exhale, follow the breath as it leaves your body. Again, how does it feel? Be aware of any sensations that you feel during each inhalation and exhalation round before beginning the exercise. Feel the expansion on the inhalation. As you exhale, feel the release of tension in your body.

If following your breath doesn't help you relax, then perhaps focusing on how your abdomen expands gently as you take a deep, slow inhale and contracts toward your spine when you release that breath may work better for you. The idea is that you find something to focus on that helps you stay mindful of each in-breath and out-breath, which then quiets your thoughts and calms your mind.

Remember, you are training your body to pay attention to sensations you probably have not been aware of before. This takes time. Frustration may set in if you expect instant results. Treat yourself with patience and kindness as you practice these new exercises. Give yourself the time *you* need to become thoroughly comfortable with this, whether it's one week or six months.

PAUSE...PAUSE AGAIN

As you become more relaxed with your breathing, begin to add a pause at the end of each inhalation and exhalation. Take a deep, slow, relaxing in-breath. At the top of the in-breath, pause before beginning the exhalation. At first, the pause may only be for a second or two. Later, as your breath becomes more relaxed and as you become more accustomed to breathing this way, you can try counting to three then four seconds while you pause your breath. This doesn't mean that you become tense as you "hold" your breath. You just pause for a few seconds and allow the "breath to breathe you" when it is ready.

This pause should feel very normal and comfortable. If at any time you feel that this stresses you and your breath becomes irregular, discontinue pausing for the time being. Sometimes when you feel very agitated and stressed, pausing may just add more stress, making you feel that you are struggling to breathe. Try pausing later when you are more relaxed and more comfortable with the exercise.

EXHALE MEANS RELAX

As you exhale, have the intension of releasing any muscle tension and relaxing your body. Begin by gently lowering your shoulders away from your ears as you begin the exhale. As your shoulders slowly move downward away from your ears, feel the wave of relaxation extend into your shoulders and your arms, causing them to feel heavy and warm. Feel the warm wave of relaxation move down through your torso. Feel your whole body loosen up as if everything inside of you has suddenly become like a wet noodle. As your body relaxes, feel the muscles in your thighs, legs, and all the way down to your tippy toes become soft, warm, and heavy.

As you inhale, feel your lungs fill with air, which adds natural buoyancy to your whole body. It's almost as if you are about to lift off and float in midair. The inhalation and exhalation work together to bring about a relaxed, warm feeling in all of your muscles.

PRACTICE AND MORE PRACTICE

It's easy as you begin any of these practices to expect quick results. When we do any of these exercises a few times or a few times a day for several days, we tend to expect to see results right away. Don't become discouraged if this isn't always the case.

Sometimes, the body adjusts very quickly to one particular exercise, and we do see the desired results very quickly. However, other times we will practice an exercise faithfully for days, maybe even weeks, and still not feel the desired calm. This is normal.

My advice is to continue doing the exercise with the intention that calm will come. Before you know it, you will feel your thoughts quiet, your mind start to calm, and your body relax. At this point, you will know that you are on your way to reaching that feeling of quietude that we all desire.

LET THE BREATH BREATHE YOU

As you practice the pause after each in-breath and out-breath, sometimes you'll find yourself so relaxed that you pause for quite a long while. As you come to the end of that long pause, you'll feel the breath begin on its own deep within you. It's almost as if you don't have to do anything except just sit quietly, and the breath will breathe all on its own.

Knowing that you are not "making" yourself breathe is a very relaxing moment. Rather, the breath started on its own without you actually doing anything to make it start. This is what I mean by "allowing the breath to breathe you." It is a very relaxing and calming moment.

ONE AT A TIME OR...ALL AT ONCE

This is such an individual consideration that I hesitate to offer any suggestions. It is absolutely up to you. However, for most people it is less stressful to start with one of the exercises within a practice at a time. This will allow you to focus on "getting it right" as far as the procedure goes. It will also establish that familiar routine, which eliminates any added stress.

This also strengthens the habit of the exercise. Repeating the exercise leads the mind and the body to accept this exercise automatically to quiet the thoughts and calm the mind. Thus, whenever you begin the exercise, your mind and your body will respond quickly to experience the peace and relaxation that you are hoping to accomplish.

Once you have become comfortable with the "how-to" of the exercise and feel that the repetitions flow effortlessly, then you are ready, if *you* feel ready, to begin the next exercise or practice. For some, just enjoying the quiet thoughts and calm mind that one exercise brings is all they feel they need at the time. So, it's important to accept the idea that whatever feels safe, comfortable, and relaxing for *you* is what is right.

SECTION 1

BREATHWORK

Breathing Exercise: Diaphragmatic Breathing
Breathing Exercise: *Ujjayi* Breath
Breathing Exercise: Left Nostril Breathing
Breathing Exercise: Alternate Nostril Breathing
Breathing Exercise: 4-7-8 Breathing
Breathing Exercise: Bumblebee Breath

BREATHWORK

OUR BREATHING IS the simplest, most natural, but most essential process in our everyday lives. We breathe 24-7 every single day of the 365 days of every year of our lives. The breath is one of the most effective tools for calming the mind and relaxing the body.

Yet, it is so often one of the most overlooked and underused ways to bring about relaxation and peace of mind. Working with our breath to calm our mind is free and effective and does not require any special equipment. Breathwork can be done anywhere at any time.

We breathe whether we are consciously aware that we are breathing or not. Since we're not aware of our breathing, an intelligence within us monitors it, making sure that we continue to breathe. Our lungs still fill with air, inhaling and exhaling regularly, whether we think about it or not.

In 1895, a German physician, Richard Kayser, first described a rather odd phenomenon. He found that we breathe through one nostril for a time, usually about two and a half hours. Then specialized tissue in that nostril swells and partially closes off that nostril. The tissue then shrinks in the other nostril, opening the airway and allowing us to breathe through that one for about two and a half hours.

This cycle then reverses, and we start all over again, breathing through the first nostril. Interestingly enough, we are not even aware that this is happening throughout the day. All we know is that we continue to inhale and exhale on a pretty regular basis.

Another interesting study published in 1994 showed that when we breathe through the right nostril, the left hemisphere of the brain is more active or dominant. Vice versa, when breathing through the left nostril, the right hemisphere of the brain is more active. This switching from one nostril to the other is done automatically by the body. It is believed that it is controlled by the autonomic nervous system.

Even though our breathing is automatic and outside of our everyday awareness, it can be controlled by our intention. This conscious awareness of our breath can help control the pattern of our breathing. We can feel more relaxed and calm when our breathing is slow, deep, gentle, and rhythmic. On the other hand, when we become agitated, our breathing is sharp and shallow.

Many of the emotions we feel have their own breathing pattern. If we are angry, our breaths come in a tight, rapid, choppy, and erratic pattern. If we are feeling stressed, our breaths come in a shallow, very fast, and hurried pattern, almost as if we don't have time to breathe. When we feel sadness, we tend to sigh, releasing the air in a slow, methodical way.

Generally, when we feel tense and anxious, our breath originates in the upper chest. As we take a breath, it feels as if we can't get a full breath to fill our lungs completely. We begin to gasp for air, what some call air hunger, trying to fill our lungs to their fullest. However, no matter how hard we try, it just doesn't feel as if we are able to take in all the air we need. Soon, we feel as if we have to gasp again just to be able to get some air into our lungs.

On the other hand, when we are relaxed, our lungs fill with air in a rhythmic, deep, easy, gentle, and steady fashion. If we pay attention to our breath, we can tell that we are calm just by observing that regular, consistent inhalation and exhalation pattern. Being aware of that calm, rhythmical rising and falling of our chest also contributes to the calmness that we feel.

It's important to add that for the best results, begin your practice of these breathing exercises at a time when you are not stressed or rushed. This gives the body and the mind the opportunity to experience the calming, quieting effects of the deep, slow, gentle breaths. If you only practice these breathing exercises when you are very stressed or nervous, it may take the body a longer time to begin to experience that feeling of calm and relaxation.

On the other hand, if you have practiced the breathing exercise during times of little or no stress, your mind and body have experienced the calming effect of the exercise. They quickly learn to respond by becoming calm, quiet, and relaxed. This soothing and relaxed feeling then becomes the reference point to return to whenever you begin to use any of the breathing exercises. Both the body and the mind will begin to calm down and relax very quickly.

That is the purpose of these breathing exercises: to become aware of the calm, deep, slow breathing in a rhythmical way that can lead to a relaxed body, quiet thoughts, and a calm mind. It's important to realize that we can help produce a relaxed, calm mind and body on demand simply by consistently making these breathing exercises a daily part of our lives. Once the body gets accustomed to breathing in a certain pattern, we can recreate those same calm and peaceful feelings on an as-needed basis.

BREATHING EXERCISES

Let's begin practicing the breathing exercises that can help calm the mind by slowing down that loop of racing thoughts. Before we begin, there is one cautionary note: if you are having trouble breathing due to asthma, a cold, or any other respiratory condition, wait until your breathing normalizes before attempting any of the breathing exercises. This advice applies to all the breathing exercises.

DIAPHRAGMATIC BREATHING

It is said that diaphragmatic breathing is the body's natural way of breathing. This breathing technique is called diaphragmatic breathing, abdominal breathing, or belly breathing. I will use the term "abdominal breathing" throughout this book.

Some people breathe this way during sleep or when very relaxed. Most of us, however, tend to breathe in a more shallow way that does not engage the abdomen in the same way as abdominal breathing. This may be due to habit, poor posture, restrictive clothing around the waist, or in some cases, conditions that may weaken the core.

So a bit of information on what the diaphragm is and how it works. The diaphragm is a dome-shaped sheet of muscle under the lungs that is instrumental in breathing. Lungs are not muscles and need help to expand and contract during breathing. This is the role of the diaphragm along with the intercostals, the muscles between the ribs.

A diaphragmatic breathing technique or abdominal breathing is one in which the diaphragm contracts on the inhale in a purposeful way and gently moves downward, away from the lungs. This allows oxygen-rich air to enter the lungs through the nose or mouth.

As the lungs fill with air, they have the room to expand fully. During the inhalation, the lower abdomen moves outward away from the spine. This allows for a full, deep breath rather than a shallow one.

During the exhalation, the diaphragm muscle expands, moving gently upward into the chest area, forcing the air that is rich in carbon dioxide out of the lungs through the nose or mouth. The lungs then release most of the air as the lower abdomen moves inward toward the spine. This results in the air, even from the lower part of the lungs, to be exhaled with each out-breath.

As you breathe out, imagine that your breath carries out all the stressful, negative, anxious feelings or thoughts like anger, fear, resentment, and sadness. Then as you breathe in, imagine that the breath is pure, energizing, and invigorating filled with pure healing energy. Continue letting go of all those heavy and negative feelings with each out-breath. Then, on the in-breath feel yourself energized and replenished with that pure healing breath. Continue this for as long as it takes you to feel refreshed and renewed.

It can be very beneficial to practice abdominal breathing until it becomes second nature to breathe this way. However, since this breathing cycle is very different from the way we breathe when stressed or anxious, it may take a little practice to become comfortable breathing this way.

When we are stressed, our inhalation usually tends to be shallow and only in the upper chest. The lower abdomen rarely expands outward with the inhale or contracts inward with the exhale. This means that the amount of air that we breathe in is less than when we allow the lower abdomen to expand outward, as in abdominal breathing.

At first, you may have to gently force your abdomen to move outward away from your spine on the inhale. This is different from what most people do even during "normal" breathing. As stated earlier, usually the chest moves in and out. The abdomen stays relatively still.

Since abdominal breathing is probably not how you are normally breathing now, your body may not know how to do it automatically. You may need to break it down into even smaller steps. Before actually beginning this exercise, practice gently moving your abdomen outward, away from your spine, on the inhale. Repeat this step over and over again until you feel comfortable doing it automatically.

Once you feel comfortable moving your abdomen outward with the inhale, then practice gently pulling your abdomen in toward the spine during the exhale. Practice this until it also feels normal. Now you are ready to put the in-and-out movement of the abdomen during the inhalation and exhalation together as a set.

You'll quickly work your way up to expanding the abdomen on the in-breath and contracting it on the out-breath without giving it a second thought. Don't worry about the diaphragm. It'll do what it's supposed to do, contract and expand, all on its own as you are breathing!

Some benefits of practicing abdominal breathing are as follows:

- Stress reduction
- Strengthening of the diaphragm
- Control of the breath
- Increased oxygenation to the body
- Increase lung capacity
- Increase sense of calm

Let's practice a few rounds of abdominal breathing:

1. Sit or lie comfortably in a quiet place where you won't be disturbed.
2. Place one hand on the chest and the other on the abdomen.
3. The hand on the chest stays still through the inhalation and exhalation.
4. Begin by inhaling slowly through the nose. The hand on the abdomen should move outward away from the spine as the abdomen expands.
5. Exhale slowly through the mouth with puckered or "pursed" lips. The hand on the abdomen moves in toward the spine as it contracts.
6. Practice this until the in-and-out movements of your abdomen with each inhalation and exhalation feel easy and natural.

This is one round of abdominal breathing. Begin with three to four rounds and slowly build up as you get more and more comfortable with this way of breathing. Remember, this is all about what feels comfortable for you. Abdominal breathing alone will help quiet your thoughts and calm your mind, and will lead to a more relaxed body.

Once you've gotten the feel for the way your abdomen moves out with the inhalation and in toward the spine with the exhalation, you don't need to use your hands anymore. You can always use your hands as a quick check, as needed, to make sure that you are doing this breathing technique correctly.

At any time throughout your day, wherever you are, whatever you are doing, return to abdominal breathing. The idea is to get to a point where it feels perfectly natural breathing this way instead of the shallow-chest way. Think of it as your default breath unless you are doing any form of exercise that requires fast breathing.

Try to incorporate abdominal breathing into all the breathing exercises as well as any of the other practices. Before long, you'll find that your body just breathes this way naturally without you having to give it any thought.

UJJAYI BREATH

To simultaneously calm your mind and energize your body, one excellent breathing technique is the ancient Yogic breathing exercise called *Ujjayi* breath, pronounced "oo-jahee." *Ujjayi* breath is often translated "victorious breath" and has been used for centuries in the Hatha Yoga practice.

Ujjayi breath is often used as a stand-alone breathing practice for calming the mind. It is known as diaphragmatic breathing, abdominal breathing, belly breathing, or deep breathing. These names all refer to the fact that the abdomen is engaged consciously in every breath, as was discussed in the previous exercise.

The sound made while practicing *Ujjayi* breath is compared to the sound of ocean waves. This rhythmic sound helps calm the mind and the body. It is described as an audible hollow, deep, yet soft hissing sound that comes from deep in your throat during the inhalation and exhalation.

The sound has also been described as the rustle of wind in the trees, or for those less poetically inclined, the sound Darth Vader made in the film *Star Wars*, only softer and gentler. As mentioned previously, if you are unfamiliar with the sound of Darth Vader's breath, many sites online will help familiarize you with that sound.

In order to hear the characteristic sound heard in *Ujjayi breath*, constrict the muscles of the upper throat on the inhale. This causes the air to rush through the constricted throat muscles, producing the sound of ocean waves. As you exhale, again constrict the throat to produce the same ocean-wave sound during the whole exhalation.

This breathing practice strengthens the diaphragm. As the diaphragm strengthens, it becomes easier to control the length and speed of the breath. This is one of the primary purposes of practicing *Ujjayi breath*. Both the inhalation and exhalation should be of the same length and through the nose.

Ujjayi breath also has numerous benefits for the entire body. Here are some of those benefits that you may enjoy by practicing it on a regular basis:

- Relieves tension, both mental and physical
- Increases oxygen flow throughout the whole body
- Helps increase mindfulness
- Helps regulate blood pressure
- Promotes a feeling of peace and tranquility
- Helps slow down the heart rate
- Helps promote relaxation
- Helps calm your mind of all the racing, swirling thoughts

Let's get started with the practice of the *Ujjayi* breath. As you will see, the actual breathing exercise is quite simple and enjoyable. Find a comfortable position, either sitting on a chair or on the floor. Be sure to wear loose-fitting clothes. Once you are comfortable with this breathing exercise, you may want to try it lying down.

As you begin this practice, try to find a time when you don't feel rushed and can dedicate at least twenty minutes to practicing *Ujjayi* breath. This allows you to feel relaxed. As your body experiences this relaxed feeling, it will associate itself with the practice of *Ujjayi* breath. Once your body has made this association, it will develop the habit and return to that relaxed state easily every time you start breathing this way.

Throughout this exercise, breathe through your nose. Give yourself the time to just sit and breathe for a short while, getting into a relaxed breathing rhythm before starting *Ujjayi* breath. Don't try to force your breath into any pattern. Just breathe normally.

Let's begin the practice of *Ujjayi* breath.

1. Sit comfortably.
2. Start to breathe gently, calmly, and naturally through your nose.
3. Throughout this exercise, breathe using the abdominal breathing technique explained earlier.
4. Inhale with the throat muscles constricted to add the soft and gentle "Darth Vader" sound during the inhalation.
5. Exhale gently, forcing the air through the constricted throat muscles, again making the soft Darth Vader sound during the exhalation.
6. Continue inhaling and exhaling with the muscles of your throat constricted, producing the soft Darth Vader sound on the inhale and exhale.

7. Each inhale and exhale is one set. At first, start out with four sets. Once comfortable with this, you can add more sets.

Throughout this breathing practice, you should hear the soft Darth Vader sound on both the inhalation and exhalation. You should continue to feel your hand on your abdomen move in toward your spine with each exhalation and out, away from your spine, with each inhalation.

It may take a little time to become comfortable inhaling and exhaling with the constricted throat muscles and, at the same time, engaging your abdomen this way, but once you have mastered this, you'll see how calming it can be. Give yourself the necessary time *for you* to feel the benefits of doing this exercise.

You can use *Ujjayi* breath whenever you are feeling overwhelmed or stressed out. To start out, it may help if you count one, two, three, four slowly as you inhale and one, two, three, four slowly on the exhale. This will help you keep each inhale the same length as the exhale. Once you are comfortable with *Ujjayi* breath, you can discontinue counting.

If you like, you can add a short pause after each inhalation and exhalation as mentioned in the "General Tips" section. This will slow down your breathing even more, adding an even greater quiet and calming effect to each round.

Begin with a short pause of a few seconds after each inhalation and exhalation. Once comfortable with that, you can start to lengthen the pause as you become more relaxed and comfortable with *Ujjayi* breath. The pause should be a natural thing. If you feel you have to strain to complete the pause, discontinue until it becomes more natural.

If at first you don't succeed, don't get discouraged. Remember that you are retraining your body in a new way of breathing. Be patient and gentle with yourself. Your body has been doing this breathing thing in a certain way, but in a very different way, for a long time. For some of us, that is a long, long, long time! Give yourself the time necessary to feel comfortable doing *Ujjayi* breath.

LEFT NOSTRIL BREATHING

This is a very easy but effective breathing exercise to use when you are feeling anxious and your mind is filled with racing thoughts. It is particularly effective when done right before going to sleep.

It is best done sitting up. You can sit on a chair or on the floor with or without cushions. It also works well to sit on your bed right before bedtime. You want to make sure that you are comfortable in order to avoid any distractions while practicing this breathing exercise.

When you feel extra tense or feel that your mind is a constant swirl of thoughts that won't settle down, this breathing technique will help quiet your mind and your body because it activates the parasympathetic nervous system. This is the "rest and relax" nervous system of the body.

Let's begin practicing the left nostril breathing exercise.

Find a comfortable, quiet spot where you won't be disturbed. Throughout the practice of left nostril breathing, you'll only breathe through the left nostril. Inhalations and exhalations should be of the same duration. If you are comfortable doing so, pause after the inhalation and exhalation for a few seconds. With time, begin to extend the pause for a longer time.

1. Extend the fingers of your right hand as if you were going to shake hands.
2. Place your right thumb gently against your right nostril, blocking the air from entering or leaving it. Now your extended fingers should be pointing upward toward the sky.
3. Begin by taking a gentle, slow, deep breath, inhaling through the left nostril. Pause.
4. Exhale gently, slowly, and completely through the left nostril. Pause.
5. Continue this cycle of inhaling and exhaling through the left nostril for seven or eight rounds or as long as you feel comfortable. It's that easy!

Each time you take a slow and deep inhale, feel your body relax as you fill your lungs with the breath of life. As you exhale, imagine a warm wave of relaxation starting at the top of your head and releasing all the stress and tension all the way to your tippy toes as the breath leaves your body. This will create a very soothing, relaxing breath cycle, which will also calm those racing thoughts and your mind.

Variation: If extending your fingers upward doesn't feel comfortable to you, try curling your fingers into your palm. Either way will bring about the same result by activating the parasympathetic nervous system.

Once you are comfortable doing the left nostril breathing exercise, you may want to extend the calming effect by adding a count.

> Inhale for a count of 1...2...3...4
> Pause for a count of 1...2...3...4
> Exhale for a count of 1...2...3...4
> Pause for a count of 1...2...3...4

ALTERNATE NOSTRIL BREATHING

Alternate nostril breathing, or *Nadi-Shodana*, as it is known in Ayurvedic medicine, has a long history for harmonizing the two hemispheres of the brain and calming the mind. It is believed that this results in a balance of physical, mental, and emotional well-being.

It also activates the parasympathetic nervous system (PSNS). This part of our autonomic nervous system controls involuntary activities in our body. When the PSNS is activated, the body is relaxed, blood pressure lowers, and the fight-or-flight response is subdued, which helps to calm and focus the mind.

Here are some of the effects on the body you may experience when you practice alternate nostril breathing:

- The practice of alternate nostril breathing benefits our hearts and lung.
- It also relaxes and calms the mind and the body.
- It reduces blood pressure.
- It increases respiratory strength and endurance.
- It improves focus and attention.
- It helps relax the muscles throughout the body.
- It increases mindfulness.
- It calms racing thoughts.

Let's get started practicing this very beneficial breathing exercise.

Sit in a comfortable chair or on the floor. Wear loose-fitting clothes so there will be no restrictions as you breathe.

1. Relax your body, and breathe naturally through both nostrils as you allow your body and mind to quiet and settle. Close your eyes if you wish.

2. Extend your index and middle finger of your right hand upward. Rest them gently on the bridge of your nose between the eyes.

3. Now bring your thumb to rest on your right nostril. Place your ring finger and your pinkie on your left nostril gently.

4. Close your eyes and begin by gently pressing your thumb against the right nostril, blocking any air from entering or escaping on that side.

5. Take a deep, slow, gentle, and smooth inhale through your left nostril.

6. Pause for a few seconds.

7. With your ring finger, close your left nostril as you release your thumb from the right nostril. Exhale through your right nostril while keeping the left one closed.

8. Pause for a few seconds.

9. Inhale through the same right nostril. Pause for a few seconds.

10. Gently close the right nostril with your thumb and release the ring and pinkie fingers from the left nostril.

11. Exhale through the left nostril while keeping the right nostril closed with your thumb.

12. Inhale deeply through the same left nostril. Pause for a few seconds.

This is one round of alternate nostril breathing. At first, do four to six of these rounds following the directions in steps six through twelve. Once you are comfortable, you can increase the number of rounds.

Once done, sit quietly with your eyes closed and enjoy how relaxed you feel. Stay here breathing through both nostrils for as long as you like, enjoying the quiet mind and relaxed body this breathing exercise induces. Remember to be gentle. Your breath is your friend.

4-7-8 BREATHING

This breathing technique is also easy to do and requires no equipment or special clothing. At first while you are learning 4-7-8 breathing, sit with a straight, relaxed back in a comfortable chair or on the floor. It is important that you keep the 4-7-8 count consistent. You can speed it up or slow it down, but keep the 4-7-8 ratio the same. With practice you will find that it becomes easier to slow the three phases down to begin inhaling and exhaling more deeply and slowly.

Place the tip of your tongue on the roof of your mouth right behind your front teeth. Keep it there throughout the entire exercise. You will be inhaling quietly through your nose, both nostrils, and exhaling through your mouth. The air will go around your tongue. Puckering or "pursing" your lips slightly may help make this less awkward.

In this exercise, you breathe in quietly through your nose and exhale forcefully through your mouth, making a "whooshing" sound. The inhalation should take less time than the exhalation. In fact, the exhalation should be slow, gentle, and relaxed so that it actually takes twice as long as the inhalation. Keep the tip of your tongue on the roof of your mouth behind your front teeth the whole time.

Let's get started.

1. Place the tip of your tongue on the roof of your mouth behind your front teeth.
2. Exhale completely through your mouth as you normally do.
3. Close your mouth. Slowly inhale through your nose to a mental count of four.
4. Hold your breath for a mental count of seven.
5. Exhale forcefully, making that whooshing sound as the air rushes out through your mouth to a mental count of eight.
6. This is one round. Begin again with the inhalation. Repeat three more times for a total of four rounds.

It is recommended that you only do four rounds when you first begin practicing 4-7-8 breathing. Once you are comfortable with four rounds, then you can gradually increase the number of rounds.

BUMBLEBEE BREATH

In Sanskrit, the name of this breathing technique is *Bhramari Pranayama*. *Bhramari* in Sanskrit literally means "bee" and *Pranayama* means "breath." Hence the name, bumblebee breath. This is a fun breathing exercise that is very calming for your body and greatly relieves mental tension to calm your mind. It's a great exercise for when you can't seem to fall asleep. The vibration produced by the bumblebee breath is credited with the soothing effect on the racing thoughts, which calms the mind.

The bumblebee breath, with its humming sound on the exhalation, extends the exhalation with a minimum of stress in a fun and relaxed way. Extending the exhalation is said to tone down your fight-or-flight response and increase your body's natural, built-in stress-relieving system, the parasympathetic nervous system.

Here's how to practice the bumblebee breath.

1. Sit comfortably on the floor or in a chair. Back is straight.
2. Gently close your eyes. Slightly tuck your chin into your chest.
3. Inhale slowly, deeply, gently, and quietly through your nose.
4. With your thumb or index finger, block your ears by gently pushing in on the outer flap between your face and your outer ear.
5. Exhale slowly, making a soft, low-pitched humming noise. Feel the vibration throughout your body.
6. Continue this breath for six to seven rounds. As you become more relaxed and comfortable with this breathing technique, you can increase the amount of rounds.

7. When you are finished with the exercise, sit quietly with your eyes closed and enjoy the relaxation that you feel.

Note: While these directions indicate to make a soft, low-pitched humming sound, try making a higher-pitched humming sound. I find that there are times when a low-pitched sound is more soothing and relaxing for my racing thoughts. At other times, a higher-pitched sound seems to calm my body and my racing thoughts more effectively. There is no right or wrong way. It's all about what works best for you at that particular time.

Variation: Once you are comfortable doing this breathing technique as described above, you may want to try this variation. Follow steps one and two above. We'll begin here with step three.

3. Inhale slowly, deeply, gently, and quietly through your nose.
4. Instead of gently holding the outer flap closed throughout the exhalation, try gently pushing it in and out quickly as you exhale.
5. Exhale slowly, making a soft or loud low-pitched humming sound.
6. Experiment with the placement of your finger on the flap to see where it is most relaxing for you.

Again, practice making low- and high-pitched sounds as you gently pushes the outer flap in and out to see which works best for you. Also, experiment with the loudness of the sound. Try pushing the flap in and out slowly, and then try by pushing it in and out more quickly for different effects. This is another example of the best way is the way it works best for *you*.

SECTION 2

MINDFULNESS

MINDFULNESS

ACCORDING TO *MERRIAM-WEBSTER*, mindfulness is defined as "The practice of maintaining a nonjudgmental state of heightened or complete awareness of one's thoughts, emotions, or experiences on a moment-to-moment basis."

As you begin practicing mindfulness, you will find that you become consciously aware of every aspect of your experience—the positive, neutral, and negative. You become aware of what you are thinking and how the thoughts are making you feel (your emotions), and you feel a heightened awareness of the experience you are going through in that moment. You also become aware of yourself and those around you with acceptance, nonjudgmental, and a newfound sense of curiosity.

Mindfulness is becoming very popular these days with many psychotherapists using it as part of their toolkit for eliminating stress and anxiety. They have found that as racing thoughts are quieted and the mind becomes calm during a mindfulness practice, the body quickly follows and relaxes.

In this busy world in which we live, our mind is constantly pulled every which way, scattering thoughts and emotions, making our mind jump from one subject to the next with no logical sequence, leaving us totally exhausted, stressed, and at times quite anxious.

Origins of Mindfulness

Mindfulness originated centuries ago as part of many ancient meditation practices. However, modern-day mindfulness is credited to Jon Kabat-Zinn, founder of the Stress Reduction Clinic at the University of Massachusetts Medical School in the late 1970s. Since then, thousands of people have found relief from a variety of conditions, including chronic pain, anxiety, racing thoughts, heart disease, sleep problems, and depression, using mindfulness as taught in the Mindfulness Stress Reduction program there.

Mindfulness or Mindlessness?

Have you ever remembered getting into the car, starting the motor, and getting on the road, but the next thing you know, you've arrived at your destination? You don't remember seeing anything along the way, stopping for red lights, or even going again when the light turned green. You don't necessarily remember what you were thinking about either. You were on automatic pilot!

Or maybe you get a bag of your favorite chips and get comfortable on the couch to watch your favorite show on TV. The next thing you know, the show is over, and the bag of chips is empty. You don't remember much of the show or how good that bag of chips tasted. Again, your thoughts were anywhere but in the present moment! You were on automatic pilot!

These are classic examples of "mindlessness" or "running on automatic pilot." Throughout both of these experiences, your mind was anywhere but where you were or on what you were doing at that moment. You could have been thinking about something that happened yesterday that upset you. Or perhaps your mind was on the long list of to-dos for tomorrow, with stress building as you tried to figure out how you were going to get it all done.

Often we are not present in our daily lives moment to moment, so we miss the subtle but good happenings in our lives. We miss out on the simple but enjoyable moments that make up our daily lives. In the above example, we completely missed how funny the main character was in the TV show or how crunchy and delicious the chips tasted!

We also miss what our body is trying to tell us. When we are running on automatic pilot, we oftentimes are not aware of the toxic "self-talk" that is on that automatic loop in our mind. We begin to feel unhappy or sad and have no idea that the thoughts we were thinking automatically are the cause for those feelings.

The human mind is notorious for dwelling on past events or trying to predict what will happen in the future based, in many cases, on what happened in the past. Some say that our brain is hardwired to do this without our necessarily being aware that we are doing it. This easily distracts us from being fully aware of what is going on in the present moment. It keeps us from living our present moment to the fullest.

Dwelling in the past also adds greatly to stress as we relive past events that we can no longer change or improve in any way. We tend to beat ourselves up over events that happened a long time ago but that in our mind seems to be happening right now. In many cases, reliving these events causes physiologic changes such as a racing heart, high blood pressure, anxious thoughts, and shortness of breath. None of these emotions or feelings is beneficial to our health.

Trying to predict future events also produces stress because we have no control over what may or may not happen. We tend to become stressed and anxious, feeling that something that didn't go well in the past will again not go well when we try it in the future. The loop of negative, disempowering thoughts just runs wildly, causing us to feel those anxious emotions.

WHAT IS MINDFULNESS?

Mindfulness is the opposite of the mindlessness we saw in the examples above. In mindfulness, we are consciously aware of and see clearly everything that is happening in our body, in our surroundings, and in our mind in the present moment. Mindfulness is paying attention to the only moment that we are alive for sure: the present moment. It's really much easier than it sounds!

Jon Kabat-Zinn, in his book *Mindfulness for Beginners*, defines mindfulness: "Mindfulness means paying attention in a particular way; on purpose, in the present moment and nonjudgmentally."[1]

Let's take a closer look at these individual components:

Paying attention in a particular way
On purpose
In the present moment
Nonjudgmentally

Paying attention in a particular way on purpose refers to our being aware consciously and purposefully of what we are doing right now, how and what we are feeling, and what is going on around us as we are doing it. This includes the thoughts we are having at that moment.

---

[1] . Jon Kabat-Zinn, *Mindfulness for Beginners: Reclaiming the Present Moment and Your* (Boulder, Colorado: Sounds True, 2016).

For example, we may be aware that we are feeling sad but not be mindful of our sadness. We may think of the feeling of sadness but immediately tell ourselves that we don't have time for this now.

Instead of pausing to take some deep, gentle breaths to determine what made us feel sad or to feel our sadness, we ignore it. Was it the poor, dirty puppy we saw on the street? Or was it because a certain woman holding a baby brought to mind the baby we have at home that isn't feeling well right now? We don't acknowledge the thoughts or situation that produced the sadness.

Let's look at vacuuming as an example. While it is a mundane activity, nevertheless, it is one most of us do on a regular basis. It lends itself quite well to mindfulness.

When we are running the vacuum mindlessly, our mind could be on a hundred different things that have nothing to do with vacuuming. We could be thinking about the upsetting discussion we had at work yesterday. Or our mind could be in the future, wondering how we are going to pay for that furnace that's about to give out.

We may be vaguely aware that we are vacuuming but not of the details of our vacuuming. We might even be talking on the phone or watching what is happening on the TV.

For example, we don't feel the vibration in our hand as we move the vacuum back and forth. We miss the pattern the vacuum makes on the rug in a crisscross fashion or the part of the rug we missed completely! We may not see that the vacuum has just picked up the earring we lost yesterday. We may not be aware of the satisfaction we feel when the job is completed. In many cases, we look at the floor but don't see much of anything, not even the vacuum.

Because we are not aware of our thoughts, they have liberty to just run loose. One thought leads to another and another and another without any rhyme or reason. We make little effort to bring our attention back to the present moment. There doesn't seem to be much purpose to the activity. However, purposefulness is very important in mindfulness.

Intending to be fully and consciously aware of the experience we are having is at the heart of mindfulness. Practicing mindfulness allows us to be aware and fully present in the moment we are experiencing. It gives us the opportunity to respond to habitual circumstances in a calmer way that may bring about desirable changes, such as lower blood pressure, a calmer mind, and a more relaxed body.

Being in the present moment encourages the mind to focus consciously on things that we are doing or are happening right now, not in the past or the future. If we don't make that conscious effort, our mind will just wander through a variety of thoughts, which also may bring a variety of emotions—anger, sorrow, regret, frustration—all produced by past memories or future worries.

We relive events that make us sad or angry and cause corresponding physical changes in our body. The past is already finished; we can't do anything about it now. While the future hasn't come yet, there is very little we can do about that. This doesn't mean that we can't think about or make plans for the future, but we do so mindfully. After all, the only time we have with certainty is the present moment.

Nonjudgmental mindfulness is perhaps the trickiest of all the components in this definition. It refers to viewing any thoughts that come into our mind with nonjudgmental in a nonreactive way. We don't just automatically classify our thoughts as good or bad. We see the event or circumstance we are thinking of as having happened—period. We may not like what happened, but we don't have to classify it as good or bad.

We observe the thought about the experience with no reaction. It happened, and we accept that it happened. We don't dwell on it or relive the experience again in our thoughts. We don't allow ourselves to get entangled in the emotions we feel when we think in detail about the experience. We notice that we are thinking about it, accept that it did happen, let it go, and watch as it leaves our mind with no judgment or feeling.

If we find ourselves feeling anger or frustration, then we acknowledge that we are having those feelings. We don't try to dismiss them or push them out of our mind by refusing to recognize that we are having the feelings. We can say something like "Oh, this experience [whatever it may be] is making me feel so angry. But it's finished, so I'll relax and let it go." This means that you don't relive the experience moment by moment again, feeling all those negative emotions for the umpteenth time.

Accepting our thoughts without judgment means that we are not resisting that something did or didn't happen. We may not be happy it happened, but we don't allow ourselves to get entangled in all the emotions and feelings that the thoughts about the situation or person produce. We sort of watch it from afar and don't allow ourselves to be taken on an emotional roller coaster of emotions one more time.

As the thought enters our mind, we don't engage in any "shouldas, couldas, or wouldas." We just think the thought and acknowledge it. Then allow it to pass on through without engaging in any thoughts, emotions, or feelings of what we should or could have done differently. We don't allow our thoughts to go down the path of what "woulda" been better or worse if we had done things differently. Any of these thoughts may lead us to emotions of anger, resentment, guilt, or shame. None of these thought patterns are beneficial to our health in any way.

Sometimes it helps us to give an emotion or feeling human characteristics. By giving it tangible characteristics, we may be able to "see" it and allow it to pass more quickly through our minds. For example, you could give the emotion a color, a shape, or a size. You could determine where it is located in your body. Then you could determine how it feels in your body. Once you've established all these characteristics, it might be easier to release that "gigantic, swirling, deep-red, funky, hot, quivering monster that's in the pit of my stomach" now.

Mindfulness is not necessarily practiced sitting quietly with your eyes closed, although it can be practiced that way too. It is a way to be fully present in your everyday life while doing everyday things. Being present mindfully allows you to consciously enjoy the moment or consciously make the decision to let an unpleasant moment pass without any anger or other negative emotion. Whatever your decision, it is made with conscious awareness. You are in control of your response.

Many studies have found that practicing mindfulness for as little as five minutes a day consistently produces many worthwhile benefits in your daily experiences. Some of these benefits may be:

- Increased ability to focus and concentrate
- Increased ability to deal with distractions
- Increased ability to manage reaction to emotional situations
- Increased empathy and compassion

- Increased ability to calm the mind
- Decreased anxiety and stress

Let's begin practicing some mindfulness exercises. As with all exercises, take a few minutes to breathe deeply, slowly, and calmly while being mindful of your breath. This allows your body to relax and your mind to center. This is a good time to incorporate abdominal breathing as described in the section on Breathwork.

MINDFULNESS EXERCISES

BREATHING MINDFULLY

Thich Nhat Hanh, one of the great modern-day mindfulness teachers, shared the following mindfulness exercise in the Zen magazine *Shambhala Sun*. He suggests that we begin practicing mindfulness by becoming consciously aware of our breathing, the most essential and natural of all life processes. Like a faithful friend, our breath is always with us.

Thay, as he is known to his students, says to pay close attention as you breathe in and as you breathe out. Breathe in slowly, gently, calmly through your nose. Pause for a second and then exhale through your mouth. Allow your mind to think only of the inhalation or exhalation you are taking in that moment.

With each inhalation and exhalation, feel wonder in the fact that you are able to breathe and the joy that you are alive and able to be aware of yourself breathing. Feel your abdomen expand and contract with each abdominal breath. Pause for a few moments after each inhalation and exhalation. Say to yourself silently, "Breathing in: I know I am alive." Repeat for the exhalation, "Breathing out: I know I am alive." Practice this for a few minutes several times throughout the day to help your awareness return to the present moment.

Even though this exercise appears to be too simple and easy to bring you into the present moment, it is amazingly effective at doing just that. Not only will it bring you into the present moment, but it will also help relax both your body and your racing thoughts. Take a few minutes right now to try it out and see how quickly and effortlessly it brings your awareness into the present moment, relaxing your body and mind.

You can practice this exercise anywhere you find yourself. You can practice it while waiting in line at the grocery store or waiting for your child's school to dismiss. If you find yourself feeling overwhelmed for any reason, just stop what you are doing, take that first inhalation, and silently say, "Breathing in: I know I'm alive." Then follow through with the exhalation. You can even add a phrase that fits the situation. For example, you could say, "I know I am alive and calm." You'll see that after a few breaths, you'll feel calmer, and those racing thoughts will have slowed down considerably.

ONE-MINUTE MINDFULNESS

This exercise is an easy one that you can do at any time wherever you are. You can do this one while standing in line at the bank, at the drive-through window, or waiting for your car to warm up before leaving home. However, this exercise is particularly beautiful and relaxing if done outside while observing nature.

Start by checking your watch to establish the time. Find an object that you can observe from where you are. If you are inside, any object small or large will do. If you are outside in nature, then find an insect, a flower, a cloud, a rock, or any object that catches your eye. Don't do anything but observe the object of your choice. Focus your eyes on it, and look at it intently. If a fly lands on the flower you are focused on, don't observe the fly. Instead, continue looking closely at the flower, noticing all the intricate, beautiful details.

Allow yourself to become totally immersed in the object. Look at it as if it is the first time you're seeing it. Observe every aspect of it as if you have to give a detailed description later on. All the while you are focused intently on this object, do so in a relaxed and harmonious way. If you feel stressed or anxious, discontinue your observation for now; the purpose of this exercise is mindful awareness to help you relax into oneness with the object.

If you spend more than one minute focusing mindfully on the object, that is perfectly fine. In fact, as you practice this exercise, you may find that you begin to lose yourself in the object. You'll also find that time goes quickly, and the minute may turn into two or three.

If for some reason, you find that you are having difficulty focusing on the object, look away. At the very beginning, as you begin the practice of this exercise, you may find that one minute is too long. That's OK. Focus for as long as you can and then try to extend the time by a few more seconds each time you practice.

As you develop your ability to focus, you'll find that it becomes easier and easier to get lost in the details of the object. And that's absolutely fine too. You'll love the feeling of wonder and awe that you begin to feel as you lose yourself in the object of your choice.

One of the greatest benefits of doing this exercise outside in nature is the calmness that results. While you are focused on the object, all those other racing thoughts seem to just go poof! You begin to feel yourself relax, and pretty soon, you are lost in the beautiful flower or the cute ladybug. You might even begin to find yourself smiling. How neat is that?

MINDFULNESS THROUGHOUT THE DAY

The title of this exercise could just as easily be, *Mindfulness Every Day, Throughout the Day*, since it includes any activity done throughout the day on a regular basis, such as brushing your teeth, pulling weeds in your garden, preparing the evening meal, or swinging your child on the playground. It's not often that we do these activities focusing our awareness on what we are doing. More often than not, we are going over our to-do list or the presentation we are about to give at work the next day, and are completely unaware of the task we are performing.

Mindfulness throughout the day is just about everything and anything we do on a daily basis. The intent of this exercise is to call attention to those daily activities that we so often do totally mindlessly but could become a source of peace and relaxation. It's amazing how an exercise this simple can give us that refreshing feeling of peace.

It can be any activity done at any time of the day. For example, brushing your teeth is something we do daily, but how often do we brush mindfully? So, to brush your teeth mindfully, begin by focusing your awareness on the toothbrush in your hand and turning the cap of the toothpaste. Be aware of the toothpaste oozing onto the brush. While putting the green or white toothpaste on the brush, appreciate the brightness or sparkling white of the color. Listen to the sound of the running water as you turn the water on to moisten the toothpaste and your toothbrush. See the water as it runs through the bristles of the toothbrush. Be aware of your hand and your arm bringing the toothbrush to your front teeth or back teeth, wherever you start brushing. Feel the foaming of the toothpaste as you begin to brush. Feel the roughness of the brush against your gums. Or feel how the toothbrush tickles the roof of your mouth. Become aware of the minty taste of the toothpaste tingling and bubbling on your tongue.

These are some suggestions, but I'm sure you get the picture! When doing these daily activities, you can be as detailed as you have time or the inclination to be. Generally, it should not take much longer to complete the activity mindfully than it normally does.

It's fun to incorporate mindfulness while doing these necessary daily activities because you can kill two birds with one stone, so to speak. You can do what needs to be done and practice your mindfulness activity at the same time without having to set aside a separate time for mindfulness. As a fringe benefit, you will have quieted your thoughts, calmed your mind, and helped your body relax. That's a win-win as far as I'm concerned!

GRATITUDE

IN *WEBSTER'S* DICTIONARY, gratitude is defined as "a feeling of thankful appreciation for favors or benefits received; warm appreciative response to kindness."

One way to define gratitude is that it is a state, a feeling of thankfulness and appreciation for the good in our lives. We recognize that the good things come to us from outside ourselves. We acknowledge that other people, those close to us or even strangers, are the givers of gifts for which we feel appreciation and gratitude. For those of a spiritual mind-set, the giver could be a higher power that is bestowing blessings on us, for which we feel deep gratitude.

Robert Emmons, who is perhaps the world's leading scientific expert on gratitude, sees gratitude as a "relationship-strengthening emotion because it requires us to see how we've been supported and affirmed by other people."[2] As we recognize that we are loved and valued by others, we feel that desire to reciprocate, to give back, or pay it forward.

WHY PRACTICE GRATITUDE?

Practicing gratitude begins by paying attention. This means that we pay attention to the everyday things that we so often aren't even aware of. By paying attention, we become mindfully aware of the moment. For example, how beautiful the white clouds look against the blue sky, or how helpful a coworker was that made your job a little easier, or how precious your child is while asleep in your arms. This can lead to uplifting feelings of thanksgiving and the desire to give back.

Hundreds of studies have been done, and they have all reached the same conclusion when it comes to the benefits of practicing gratitude. The research conducted by Robert Emmons suggests that these benefits can be enjoyed by all people who practice gratitude regardless of the adversity a person is going through in life. Some of the people, ages eight to eighty, in the studies have been elderly facing death, women facing breast cancer, both men and women dealing with progressive muscular conditions, and parents dealing with the loss of children.

---

[2] . Robert Emmons, *Gratitude Works!: A 21-Day Program for Creating Emotional Prosperity* (San Francisco, Ca: Jossey-Bass, 2013).

Gratitude has been found to be one of the most reliable ways of increasing happiness and satisfaction with life. In studies done by Emmons and his colleague, Mike McCullough, they found that practicing gratitude strengthens the immune system, lowers blood pressure, makes us feel better when we are sick, and inspires us to take better care of our health in general.

Here are some of the top research-based benefits for your mind, body, and spirit attributed to practicing gratitude:

- Practicing gratitude also relieves anxiety and stress. It has been found helpful in relieving PTSD in some cases.
- People who practiced gratitude regularly slept better, spent less time awake during the night, and woke up feeling more refreshed. Perhaps for those who don't practice gratitude, the advice should be to count your blessings instead of those sheep!
- Gratitude encourages people to forgive themselves even after a bitter divorce or other traumatic turn of events.
- People who feel gratitude are more likely to "pay it forward," even to strangers they have never met before. Gratitude makes people more optimistic, altruistic, willing to give, and compassionate.
- It helps them feel more outgoing so they enjoy life more, therefore, feeling less lonely and isolated.

- People who practice gratitude experienced more joy and happiness in their lives.
- Those practicing gratitude seem to experience less stress.

Now that we are aware of the many benefits that we can experience practicing gratitude, let's delve into some simple but very effective ways to practice gratitude while quieting our thoughts and calming the mind.

The first exercise doesn't require any special equipment, nor does it need to be done at a certain time or place. If you wish, set aside a time dedicated to recognizing all the things to be grateful for. Another way is to go throughout your day looking for things to be grateful for. This makes for a very uplifting way to spend a day!

GRATITUDE EXERCISES

MINDFULNESS GRATITUDE

Many of us spend a great amount of time seeing only what we want to see in our lives. Others tend to think the same thoughts over and over again, never really being aware that the loop is continually running. Some give a greater importance to negative aspects of their lives, which gives them a distorted sense of reality. Gratitude is a helpful practice to stop these negative thought patterns.

Studies have shown that the mind cannot focus on negative thoughts at the same time it is focusing on positive thoughts. As you begin to focus on all the things and people in your life that you feel gratitude for, all those negative thoughts are gently but steadily pushed out of your mind. The result is that your thoughts begin to quiet and your mind feels the calm that you are searching for.

Begin this exercise by taking in a deep inhalation and saying to yourself silently the words of Thich Nhat Hahn as explained in the Breathwork section: "Breathing in: I know I am alive." Then on the exhalation, "Breathing out: I know I am alive." To add another layer of relaxation, use abdominal breathing with each inhalation and exhalation. Continue this for a few minutes, feeling an easing of any tension and stress as your mind becomes calm and your body relaxes.

Now begin to reflect on a feeling of gratitude for all the things you are blessed with that so often are taken for granted, such as your breath. From the air that you breathe daily without giving this process a second thought, to the car that you drive that gets you to and from all your daily travels, to the loving and caring relationships that bring you such deep and loving moments, any of these are bound to inspire deep gratitude.

Think of the abundance of food that is available to you. Think of all the different stores and merchants that supply you with whatever you could possibly need or want. Think of all the people involved in the planting, cultivating, processing, packaging, and selling of that abundant supply of food. Feel deep gratitude for all they do to contribute to your well-being.

We have all been given the deepest blessing of all: the gift of life. Along with that gift, we have family, friends, coworkers, and relatives. We have the gift of good health and the possibility of helping others that are in the process of recovering theirs. We have the gift of our senses, which help us know and enjoy the abundance that is available to us in our lives. As we go through our day mindfully, we have the opportunity to focus on our blessings. This gives us the opportunity to feel gratitude for so many things.

This feeling of gratitude gives calmness to our thoughts. It's very difficult to be thinking of how bad things are in our lives when we are thinking of how much is right with our lives. Continue throughout the day focusing on your blessings to find things to be grateful for.

At first, you may need to make an effort to stop what you are doing to think about the abundance that you feel gratitude for. That is perfectly normal. This is something new for your mind to focus on. Once your mind becomes accustomed to finding things to be grateful for, it will be easier to find both the time to think about gratitude and things for which to be grateful.

As Meister Eckhart tells us, if the only prayer we ever say is "thank you," we have said enough. Remember to focus on blessings and feel the warm, loving gratitude for a rich and blessed life. Allowing the attitude of gratitude to become your focus makes for a life well lived, appreciated, and enjoyed.

GRATITUDE JOURNAL

This exercise is an extension of the previous one but with benefits all of its own. The many things you are grateful for feel more real if you take the time to write them down. Where you write your entries is up to you. It can be as simple as a spiral-bound notebook or as fancy as a leather-bound journal.

You can start by writing three to five things in your journal on a daily basis. Then continue to add more as you become more focused on finding things that you feel gratitude for throughout your day. With the intention of looking for things to be grateful for, you'll find that you begin to see all the many things, big and small, that otherwise you may have overlooked. It's a great feeling as you go through your day to find something that you know will make its way into your journal as that day's entry.

A journal also gives you the opportunity to go back and reread entries made previously. It's a nice way to see how your gratitude expands to encompass many different areas of your life. Often when you go back to reread your entries, you'll find that at first the entries were mostly of material things. However, as time goes on, your entries may become more spiritually based.

For example, at the beginning you may have an entry about how grateful you are for your car that starts faithfully every morning or how grateful you feel for having the time to make your favorite dish for dinner. Later on, your entries may be more about the gratitude you feel for the time spent laughing and talking with your best friend or the deep gratitude you feel as you hold your healthy and happy child in your arms.

One huge benefit of keeping a gratitude journal is that it becomes a way of tracking your happiness. As you are writing the things you feel gratitude for, you can't help but feel that warm, fuzzy feeling of happiness about all the blessings in your life. You become more aware of and begin to appreciate all the good things, big and little, that you experience in your daily life. Things you so often take for granted.

As your thoughts are on gratitude and happiness, they can't be on stress and anxiety because the two kinds of thoughts are mutually exclusive. Spending time feeling gratitude will help quiet the anxious thoughts and calm your mind. It will increase feelings of love and appreciation along with the realization of all the good in your life.

There is no best time to write your gratitude entries in your journal. Some prefer to do it first thing in the morning. Others review their day in the evening, writing all the people, events, conversations, and so on that they feel gratitude for. Either way, you'll feel that warm, loving feeling of gratitude for a blessed life.

Again, the entries in the journal can be as short as one word or as long as several paragraphs. It all depends on the amount of time you have and on how much you want to write. Usually people write a few words that will help them identify and remember the details of the entry when they come back to it several weeks, months, or years later.

AUTOGENIC TRAINING OR AUTOGENIC RELAXATION

Autogenic Relaxation Exercise

AUTOGENIC TRAINING OR AUTOGENIC RELAXATION

Dr. Johannes Heinrich Schultz first developed the relaxation technique in the 1920s and named it Autogenic Training. Since it was easy to learn, very effective in reducing stress, and relatively inexpensive to teach to groups, Autogenic Training or Autogenic Relaxation, as it is also called, spread quickly throughout Europe as well as Asia, and finally came to the United States. I will refer to it is Autogenic Relaxation.

In the 1970s, Dr. Herbert Benson, an American cardiologist who founded the Mind-Body Medical Institute in Massachusetts General Hospital in Boston, Massachusetts, introduced autogenic relaxation into his list of calming techniques. The use of these techniques produced what he called the "relaxation response" in his patients.

Presently, there have been over three thousand clinical studies showing the effectiveness of autogenic relaxation in healing disease, treating psychological conditions, promoting general well-being, managing stress, calming the anxious mind, making decisions, solving problems, and enhancing creative thinking.

Autogenic Relaxation Explained

Autogenic relaxation silently "talks" you through a series of sensation phrases that calm down the sympathetic nervous system, which is the fight-or-flight part of our central nervous system. Once this system is calm, then the parasympathetic nervous system, the rest-and-relax part of the central nervous system, is turned on to help the muscles relax and the mind feel calm.

Autogenic relaxation is a mind-body form of relaxation in which your mind can influence your body, bringing about changes in blood pressure, heart rate, circulation, and calming the mind. It is, therefore, a therapy taught to a person, for that person's use, to calm the mind or relieve stress. You carry out this process for yourself, by yourself, in order to help yourself.

This relaxation exercise is usually done either sitting in a comfortable chair or lying in bed. It is particularly effective in inducing sleep, so a good time to practice this exercise is right before going to sleep.

Autogenic relaxation is not a form of talk therapy. The phrases that are repeated throughout the exercise are said silently, in your mind. It is often helpful to pair slow, deep inhalations and exhalations, as in abdominal breathing, with the repetition of the phrases. For example, breathe in slowly and deeply as you say silently to yourself, "My arms are heavy and warm." On the slow, deep exhalation, silently say, "I'm at peace." Instead of "I'm at peace," you could say, "I'm completely calm."

As you are saying the various phrases, add the element of mindfulness. Release all thoughts that may be stressful. Think of nothing else except what the phrase is telling you. Use your imagination to feel the warmth and heaviness of your arms or the coolness of your forehead as you repeat the phrases silently. This passive concentration helps you calm your thoughts and relieve that stressed-out mind. In the process, your muscles relax and your body feels calm.

If during an autogenic relaxation session, you find yourself crying or becoming emotional, that's a common occurrence. Again, practice what we learned in mindfulness. Feel the emotion without judging it. Allow the emotion that is produced by the thought to pass through you without becoming involved or chasing it. However, if you become too stressed, stop the exercise. Return to it when you feel more calm and ready to begin again.

The benefits you may enjoy when you practice autogenic relaxation on a consistent, regular basis are many. You may experience the following changes:

- You sleep more soundly and feel more relaxed upon waking.
- There is a slowing of the heart rate.
- It may become easier to deal with the daily stresses of life.
- You react more calmly to daily happenings that you can't control.
- There is a lowering of blood pressure.
- You feel more relaxed throughout the day.
- You experience a feeling of warmth and relaxation in your body.

Let's begin practicing autogenic relaxation.

Remember to say the phrases silently in your mind. As you say the phrases silently, focus on feeling the sensations of warmth, heaviness, coolness, or relaxation each phrase is describing. Practice mindfulness to focus only on the words and sensations of the phrases.

This is an excellent time to practice abdominal breathing to add another layer of calm to the practice. On the in-breath, your stomach expands as you say silently to yourself the sensation phrase. On the out-breath, it contracts as you silently say, "I'm at peace."

Find a comfortable position either sitting or lying down. Preferably, keep your arms and legs resting comfortably but not touching any other part of your body. You may find soft, quiet, and relaxing background music helpful. Experiment with this.

Say each sensation phrase six times. Each time follow the sensation phrase with "I'm at peace."

For example:

On the in-breath, your stomach expands as you silently say and feel, "My right foot and leg are heavy and warm."

On the out-breath, your abdomen contracts toward your spine as you silently say, "I'm at peace."

Autogenic Relaxation Exercise

Autogenic Relaxation Script

Before beginning the Autogenic Relaxation sets, take a few deep, slow breaths to quiet your mind and center yourself. If you are comfortable doing so, incorporate abdominal breathing as described in the breathwork section into the exercise. Also, become mindful throughout the exercise by focusing on feeling the sensations in the phrases. Adding these two practices quiets the thoughts and calms your mind by adding several layers of relaxation used together.

Here is a sample script that you could use as a starter script.

Set 1: (Repeat six times)
In-breath: My right hand and arm are heavy and warm.
Out-breath: I'm at peace.

Set 2: (Repeat six times)
In-breath: My left hand and arm are heavy and warm.
Out-breath: I'm at peace.

Set 3: (Repeat six times)
In-breath: My right foot and leg are heavy and warm.
Out-breath: I'm at peace.

Set 4: (Repeat six times)
In-breath: My left foot and leg are heavy and warm.
Out-breath: I'm at peace.

Set 5: (Repeat six times)
In-breath: My arms and hands are heavy and warm.
Out-breath: I'm at peace.

Set 6: (Repeat six times)
In-breath: My legs and feet are heavy and warm.
Out-breath: I'm at peace.

Set 7: (Repeat six times)
In-breath: My heartbeat is calm and regular.
Out-breath: I'm at peace.

Set 8: (Repeat six times)
In-breath: My abdomen is soft and warm.
Out-breath: I'm at peace.

Set 9: (Repeat six times)
In-breath: My forehead is cool and relaxed.
Out-breath: I'm at peace.

Set 10: (Repeat six times)
In-breath: My breathing is deep and regular.
Out-breath: I'm at peace.

Set 11: (Repeat six times)
In-breath: My thoughts are quiet and calm.
Out-breath: I'm at peace.

Set 12: (Repeat six times)
In-breath: My whole body is heavy and warm.
Out-breath: I'm at peace.

Once you have gone through all the sets, stay here breathing quietly and deeply for as long as you like. Enjoy this wonderful feeling of complete and total relaxation. Your arms and legs will truly feel warm and heavy. Your heartbeat will certainly be calm and regular. Your thoughts will be quiet and calm. Your whole body will be warm, heavy, and relaxed. And, if a smile comes to your lips, that is absolutely perfect!

Sometimes it may happen that you complete all the rounds and you still feel tense and unable to relax. In that case, I usually just go back to the beginning of the exercise and repeat all the rounds. It seems that the first complete set is needed to begin the relaxation process in the body. The second time around actually relaxes the muscles, and you begin to feel your mind calm and the body relax.

Feel free to change the order of these sets to create your own. The feeling words are also interchangeable. For example, you can say, "My thoughts are relaxed and free."

You can also design your own Autogenic Relaxation script by adding other parts of your body. Here are some examples:

My feet (hips, ankles, toes, knees) are heavy and warm.
My shoulders (neck, face, jaw, eyes, chin) are warm and relaxed.

Once you have practiced the long form of autogenic relaxation for a while and are reaping the benefits, you can use a shortened version with good results. Your body will respond to the shortened version as well as the longer version once you have "trained" it to relax when it hears the words and feels the sensations happening in the body.

Again, you can use any of the sets that are important to you or you can use the version I've provided below.

Shortened Autogenic Relaxation Script

Set 1: (Repeat six times)
In-breath: My arms and hands are heavy and warm.
Out-breath: I'm at peace.

Set 2: (Repeat six times)
In-breath: My legs and feet are heavy and warm.
Out-breath: I'm at peace.

Set 3: (Repeat six times)
In-breath: My heartbeat is calm and regular.
Out-breath: I'm at peace.

Set 4: (Repeat six times)
In-breath: My abdomen is soft and warm.
Out-breath: I'm at peace.

Set 5: (Repeat six times)
In-breath: My breathing is deep and regular.
Out-breath: I'm at peace.

Set 6: (Repeat six times)
In-breath: My whole body is relaxed and warm.
Out-breath: I'm at peace.

Once you have practiced the relaxation sets and are comfortable with them, visualize yourself in a favorite relaxing scenario. Maybe you see yourself lying on a warm, sunny beach feeling all the sensations in your body as you relax and distress. As you say each set, feel the rays of the sun on the parts of the body warming and relaxing them.

Perhaps your favorite place is in the woods with a babbling brook nearby where you feel the mist all around you and hear the sound of the water. That will work too. Again, this is all about *you* and what works best for *you*. There is no right or wrong scenario.

Autogenic relaxation takes time to master. Be patient and gentle with yourself. Give yourself the necessary time to feel these sensations in your body. Some recommend that you practice each set for one week, several times a day, before moving on to the next set.

If you find that doing all the ten sets listed above at the beginning of your practice is too much, start with two or three. Choose the first two or three sets and begin with those. Then, add other sets as you become more comfortable. Remember that everyone responds in his or her own time to these exercises. Give yourself the time *you* need to realize the calmness that you are seeking.

Meditation

MEDITATION

ANY BOOK ON techniques and practices to quiet racing thoughts and calm the mind would not be complete without a section on meditation. While the scope of this book does not allow for an in-depth study of meditation and the different kinds of meditation, it does allow for an introduction. An Internet search will yield many avenues to explore for detailed information on meditation.

WHAT IS MEDITATION?

Meditation is the practice of training your attention to concentrate on a single focal point, such as concentrating on the breath or on a word, called a mantra. Another kind of meditation is guided meditation, which is done with the help of a guide, either one-on-one or in a group. This guide can be a video, a written script, or a meditation teacher.

How long you meditate is entirely up to you. Meditating for just five minutes in the morning and evening will yield noticeable results in focus, calmness, and even improve sleep. Generally, it is recommended that you meditate for twenty minutes twice a day. Deepak Chopra has said that he meditates daily in the morning for four hours! No one is saying that everyone should do that, but if after a while you can extend your meditation beyond the twenty minutes, you can rest assured that the benefits you will experience will multiply exponentially!

Meditation is a good practice that helps you start your day with quiet thoughts, a calm and focused mind, and a relaxed body. By the same token, it's a great way to end your day, leading to restful and relaxing sleep. Again, this is something to experiment with. Start out with a few minutes once or twice a day. Then build slowly to twenty minutes and allow the next step to evolve with time and practice.

Meditation has been practiced around the world for centuries. It has been a part of many religious and spiritual groups, especially in the Eastern cultures, staying mainly in Asia. It made its way to the United States in the 1960s and 1970s. It is now practiced around the world with many health benefits, such as reducing stress, quieting thoughts, stilling the mind, and relaxing the body.

There are many different kinds of meditation. Buddhism teaches that meditation is the practice that is the foundation for the cultivation of a calm, still, and positive state of mind. This practice is done in silence in order to withdraw the attention from any outward sensory stimuli. This allows the mind to go inward, and as thoughts quiet, the mind becomes peaceful and still.

Chinese meditation emphasizes living in harmony with nature. The main purpose is to quiet the thoughts and calm the body and mind in order to find inner peace by unifying body and spirit. As the body quiets, the mind follows, and the result is a peaceful and calm feeling throughout body and mind.

Taoist meditation observes the natural laws of change in the world around us. The focus of those practicing this kind of meditation is to align themselves with the wisdom and power of these laws to become one with their source. Because of this unity, thoughts quiet, the mind becomes still and calm, and the body relaxes. This feeling of oneness produces general happiness and well-being throughout the mind and body.

These are only three of the many kinds of meditation, but the one common thread running through all meditation types is the quieting of thoughts and calming of the mind, which promotes a relaxed body. Once this state is achieved, an overall sense of well-being and joy is sure to follow. Among the long-term benefits a regular Meditation practice provides are reducing stress, releasing worrying thoughts, and coping with illness.

The beauty of meditation is that there are many different and wonderful ways of practicing. Walking Meditation is practiced outside when you go for a walk. It can be practiced as you walk in a park, on a beach, or around the block where you live. Some call it mindful walking meditation because as you are walking slowly, you are mindfully aware of what is happening within and around you.

Breath Awareness Meditation is another way to practice and one we will explore in this book. During this meditation, you are only mindful of every in-breath and every out-breath. Your mind focuses its awareness on each inhale and exhale. This is a very simple yet effective way to quiet your thoughts, calm your mind, and help your body relax. It is also a good first experience with meditation.

Because your mind is focused on the in-breath and out-breath, it does not wander as easily following every thought that comes along. If you find that your mind is following a thought, gently bring it back to focus on the breathing. I usually add abdominal breathing to this exercise. This makes it easy for my mind to stay focused by following the expansion and contraction of my abdomen.

MANTRAS

You can easily add a mantra to your meditation practice. A mantra is a word that you say silently, to yourself, while you focus on the inhalation and exhalation of each breath. Saying a mantra gives your mind something to think about while you meditate. "Om or Aum" is one of the traditional mantras.

Another often-used mantra is "So Hum." In Sanskrit the words mean, "I Am." However, "love," "peace," or any other word that feels right for you will help you focus. As you inhale, you can say the full mantra, "So Hum" or "peace." Then on the exhale, you can repeat the same full mantra.

It's also very calming to stretch out the word to follow each inhalation and exhalation. For example, as you slowly begin the inhale, silently say the mantra, but stretch it out to throughout the whole inhale "peeeeeaace." Then, on the exhale, follow this same pattern to the end of the breath. You could also say one mantra on the inhale, "peeeeeaace" and another one on the exhale, "loooooove."

When using the "So Hum" mantra, you would stretch out the "Soooooo" throughout the inhale and "Huuuummmm" to the end of the exhale. If using the "Om or Aum" mantra, stretch the "Auuummmm" sound with each inhale and exhale. Try these all out until you find the one that resonates with you perfectly. That one will bring you the most peace. I find that using the Sanskrit mantras helps me focus better because the words don't have any special meaning, which might trigger a thought. In this way, I eliminate any distraction that might interrupt my focus.

Studies on meditation have concluded that it calms the mind by calming the sympathetic nervous system, which as explained in part one, is responsible for the fight-or-flight response. Meditating eliminates the loop of anxious, repetitive thoughts that lead to anxiety. A regular meditation practice enhances the parasympathetic nervous system (PNS) and the rest-and-relaxation response. This in turn calms the amygdala, quiets the anxious thoughts, and calms the mind.

Let's begin our meditation practice with a Breath Awareness Meditation. This meditation is similar to the Mindful Breathing exercise in the mindfulness section of this book. It is stressed here because of its effectiveness in calming the mind and relaxing the body.

MEDITATION EXERCISES

BREATH AWARENESS MEDITATION

Sit either on the floor or on a chair with a straight but relaxed back. Try not to lean into the back of the chair. If you are comfortable sitting in the cross-legged position, do so. However, if this is uncomfortable in any way, just sit where and how you feel most comfortable.

Sometimes, at the beginning of the practice of meditation, it helps to focus on the expanding and contracting of the abdomen with each inhalation and exhalation as mentioned earlier. Once you become more relaxed and comfortable with the exercise, then turn your focus to the sensations of your breath alone.

Once you have practiced this meditation and feel relaxed, add the mantra of your choice. If you're not sure which one to start with, choose "love" or "peace." Then, try the Sanskrit mantras to see which one feels more soothing to you. You will quickly "feel" the one that is right for you.

1. Close your eyes and take a few deep, natural breaths to center yourself. Become mindfully aware of any sounds, thoughts, feelings, or physical sensations.
2. Breathe through both nostrils without trying to control the breath.
3. Feel the sensation as your breath enters and leaves your nose. Continue to focus only on each breath.
4. If your mind wanders, gently bring it back to focus again on your breath. Let your thoughts come and go without becoming engaged in them.
5. Continue in this way, focusing on the sensations with each in-breath and out-breath.

At first, it may seem that the mind is even busier with more thoughts than before you began the meditation. In reality, what is happening is that you are becoming aware of all the thoughts that are usually in your busy monkey-mind!

You may feel tempted to follow all those thoughts, but this temptation must be resisted because this is not the purpose of the meditation. Instead, return your focus to the sensations of your inhale and exhale without engaging any of the thoughts. In a way, you are also practicing mindfulness by being in the present moment as you inhale and exhale, instead of following your every thought.

If you find that you do follow any of the thoughts, and this will happen, no need to worry. Just return your focus to the sensations of breathing in and out. Do this as many times as it takes to return your focus to each in-breath and out-breath. Soon you'll find that the mind begins to quiet and becomes more and more calm.

Once you are comfortable with saying the mantra, you can pair saying the mantra with focusing on the movement of the abdomen by adding abdominal breathing. However, if you find that it is too much to focus on the two at the same time, just begin with the one you feel most comfortable doing. You can always add the other later on.

By practicing this meditation for ten to fifteen minutes on a daily basis, you will find that your mind becomes calmer and feels refreshed. Your stress level will be greatly reduced. You'll find yourself feeling more relaxed and better able to cope with everyday situations and concerns.

BREATH COUNTING MEDITATION

Breath Counting meditation is similar to Breath Awareness meditation, but with a simple add-on. It is a deceptively easy, but very effective meditation to quiet thoughts for a calm mind. Sit with a straight back on a chair, on the floor, or on the bed wherever you are most comfortable. Gently close your eyes. Take a few deep breaths allowing yourself to breathe naturally without influencing the depth or the rhythm of the breath.

Step 1: Take a deep breath. As you exhale, count "one" silently to yourself.

Step 2: Continue breathing, count "two" on the next exhalation.

Step 3: Continue counting on each exhalations until you reach "ten."

Step 4: Once you reach "ten" begin a new round counting "one" on the next exhalation.

Count only on the exhalations. The count should never go above "ten." However, don't be surprised if you find yourself counting to "12" or "20" or maybe even "30!" This will let you know that your mind and attention have wandered. At this point, just begin a new round by starting the count at "one" again.

As you begin this practice, start by counting the breath for 5-10 minutes. As you become more comfortable, you can increase the amount of time. Don't become frustrated if you aren't able to count to ten on each round. Give your mind time to adjust and become more disciplined. Everyone is different and has a different learning curve. You will find that this exercise will help you quiet your thoughts and relax your mind.

Here is a simple twist to try when you are able to count to "ten" easily without becoming distracted. Once you have reached "ten", begin to count backwards to "one." On the next exhalation, you would count "nine" and so on until you reached "one" again. This would complete one round.

Again, experiment with this. Begin by doing a few rounds. Once you are comfortable, then you can add more rounds. This meditation exercise is a great way to keep your mind focused, therefore, quieting your thoughts to achieve a calm mind.

LOVING-KINDNESS MEDITATION

One kind of meditation from the Buddhist tradition is the Loving-Kindness Meditation or *metta* Meditation. The word *metta* means kindness, goodwill, benevolence, and loving-kindness. This meditation is said to open the heart to love and compassion.

As your mind focuses on accepting warm, loving feelings of compassion toward yourself and others, it tends to block out any anxious thoughts. The mind is not capable of focusing on love and compassion while focusing on worrisome or fearful thoughts at the same time. As you focus on loving, compassionate thoughts, the result will be the exclusion of fearful, worrisome thoughts leading to a quiet, calm mind.

This exercise is used to promote warm feelings of acceptance and love to oneself, others, and the whole universe. It is said that Loving-Kindness Meditation (LKM) can open and "sweeten" the mind, producing calm thoughts of acceptance and compassion toward oneself and others. LKM first teaches the one practicing to love and accept himself or herself. Then it moves on to encourage the same feelings for all other beings living in the world.

Hundreds of scientific studies have been conducted as to the benefits of meditation. The conclusion is that most types of meditation offer similar benefits when practiced regularly. Some of the benefits of meditation in general, and LKM in particular, are as follows:

- Fewer troublesome, recurring thoughts
- Less fear and anxiety
- Increased feelings of connectedness and compassion
- Enhanced self-esteem and self-acceptance
- Increased feelings of gratitude and love
- Decreases depression and loneliness
- Reduced blood pressure and improved heart rate
- Strengthened mental focus and concentration

Let's begin practicing LKM. While there may be variations to this traditional approach, most practitioners agree on this sequence for LKM. Here are the steps in the traditional LKM sequence.

Begin by extending:

> Loving-kindness to yourself
> Loving-kindness to a special or beloved friend, family member, or teacher
> Loving-kindness to a neutral person, a stranger, or someone you don't know well
> Loving-kindness to someone you find difficult
> Loving-kindness to everyone in the universe

During your practice of LKM, many added techniques will enhance your meditation. Visualize yourself and your friend or teacher smiling warmly and/or embracing. Imagine that they are sitting with you. Take the time to experience the warm loving-kindness that you feel at the time of this interaction. Feel the warmth within you as you extend love and kindness to the other person.

Another way is to reflect on a positive attribute about you or the others mentioned. Think about what they may have done to show they cared for you or what you may have done that showed they were special to you. Use softly spoken words such as "I send you loving-kindness now." Use any and all ways to increase that loving-kindness feeling toward yourself and the others in your meditation.

To practice LKM, find a quiet place where you'll not be disturbed. Sit comfortably with your eyes closed, either on the floor or in a chair. Start by taking a few deep, slow, gentle abdominal breaths to center yourself. Settle into the slow pattern of your breathing for a while. Release all tension and worries of the day as you mindfully feel your breath.

Become mindful of how you are feeling, of any sensations in your body, of thoughts you are having, or of any discomfort you may be feeling. In other words, practice mindfulness. By beginning the exercise with mindfulness, you are gently acknowledging any anxious thoughts you may be having. If there is a thought or a sensation that is particularly insistent or strong, allow yourself to accept that it is there. Then, tell yourself that you will deal with it later, after the meditation. Continue breathing.

Close your mind to any thoughts of yesterday or tomorrow, focusing your attention only on the present moment and your breath. As the stress-filled thoughts are released, your thoughts will begin to quiet, the mind will become calm, and your body will begin to relax also. Continue breathing this way until you feel ready to start.

Step 1: Begin extending loving-kindness to yourself by saying the following:

> ➢ May I be filled with loving-kindness.
> ➢ May I be safe from all dangers.
> ➢ May I be happy and loved.

➤ May I be well in mind and body.
➤ May I be peaceful and at ease.

This is the first step in the practice of LKM. The most important thing at this point is to develop that loving, kind, and accepting feeling toward yourself. Practice as often as you like until you feel the warmth, love, and compassion the words convey toward yourself.

Don't be discouraged if at first the words sound mechanical or hollow. Be kind to yourself. Give yourself time to develop that loving-kindness and compassion toward yourself before continuing on with the rest of the meditation.

It may take some time before you feel ready to extend loving-kindness to someone else. That's perfectly fine. We are all different, and taking the time you need is so important. Be kind, patient, gentle, and loving toward yourself during this part of the meditation.

Once you begin to feel loving-kindness toward yourself, then you can move on to extending it to someone loved by and special to you. It can be a relative, parent, friend, teacher, pastor, or anyone that is special to you. Keep that person in mind as you repeat the phrases with loving feeling.

Begin by taking a few minutes to extend loving-kindness to yourself using the script provided above. Then go on by using these same phrases while thinking of the person who is loved by or special to you. In your heart, feel your appreciation and loving-kindness for the special person you've chosen as you begin the next step of this meditation.

Step 2: Extend loving-kindness to a special or beloved friend, family member, or teacher

> ➢ May you be filled with loving-kindness.
> ➢ May you be safe from all dangers.
> ➢ May you be happy and loved.
> ➢ May you be well in mind and body.
> ➢ May you be peaceful and at ease.

Continue to express loving-kindness to this special person in your life. Expressing gratitude helps encourage feelings of love for that person, as a benefactor, as well as for you, the receiver. It strengthens feelings of being connected, appreciated, and loved.

Stay on step two as long as you wish. The longer you do steps one and two, the more loving-kindness you'll feel toward yourself as well as toward the other person. Once you experience that strong loving and caring feeling toward yourself and the other person, you are ready for the next step.

Now you are ready to practice LKM with the same phrases, only this time they'll be directed toward a neutral person. This can be someone you are acquainted with but don't know very well. It can be someone you see often in a store, a nurse, a coworker, your doctor, or perhaps a neighbor. Say the same phrases while sending him or her loving-kindness for happiness, safety, and love.

Begin by saying the phrases for yourself and for a special loved person, feeling that loving-kindness well up in your heart. Then go on to step three, keeping in mind the neutral person you have chosen. Try to feel that warm, caring feeling even though you don't know this person well at all. Remember that everyone deserves to feel loved, happy, and safe even if you don't know them very well.

Step 3: Extend loving-kindness to a neutral person, a stranger, or someone you don't know well.

> ➢ May you be filled with loving-kindness.
> ➢ May you be safe from all dangers.
> ➢ May you be happy and loved.
> ➢ May you be well in mind and body.
> ➢ May you be peaceful and at ease.

Stay on step three as long as you like. Always begin with step one and continue through the steps. This allows you to learn the phrases well and allows you to expand your loving-kindness to yourself and others.

Now you're ready to expand your loving-kindness beyond just loved ones or neutral people to someone whom you consider a difficult person. Perhaps the relationship with this person has been hurtful or produced anger. Try to release any resentment or anger toward this person. Focus on seeing that he or she also has feelings or moments of uncertainty or perhaps is going through difficult times. Remind yourself that this person also feels pain and anxiety and is deserving of love, happiness, compassion, and kindness.

Begin by going through steps one through three. Now say the same phrases with a warm, open, and compassionate heart while directing loving-kindness to that difficult person. Again, stay in this step as long as you like.

Step 4: Extend loving-kindness to someone you find difficult

> ➤ May you be filled with loving-kindness.
> ➤ May you be safe from all dangers.
> ➤ May you be happy and loved.
> ➤ May you be well in mind and body.
> ➤ May you be peaceful and at ease.

This final step allows your awareness and loving-kindness to extend out in all directions beyond yourself, a loved one, a neutral person, and a difficult one to all beings on the planet. Those living in richness or sadness, poverty or abundance, war or peace are all included in your loving-kindness. Acknowledge that all beings experience joy and sadness. Recognize that all beings want and deserve love, happiness, and kindness shown to them just as you do. Feel your heart open as you extend to them these warm and loving feeling filled with love and compassion.

Step 5: Extend loving-kindness to everyone in the universe

> ➤ May all beings be filled with loving-kindness.
> ➤ May all beings be safe from all dangers.
> ➤ May all beings be happy and loved.
> ➤ May all beings be well in mind and body.
> ➤ May all beings be peaceful and at ease.

Now close the practice by extending loving-kindness to yourself again using the same phrases. Sit in silence for as long as you like to experience the feelings of loving-kindness that have been generated. Appreciate the love that is generated toward all these people through this meditation. Loving-Kindness Meditation is one of the most satisfying practices you can engage in.

If you find that time is an issue but would like to practice a shortened version of Loving-Kindness meditation, go through the script as it is written below. You would extend loving-kindness to yourself, then go right into extending it to the special person, then to the neutral person, and so on to complete the meditation. Be sure to take a few minutes to center yourself by breathing slowly and gently before beginning the actual meditation.

Here is the whole script for the Loving-Kindness Meditation:

For yourself:

> ➤ May I be filled with loving-kindness.

- ➢ May I be safe from all dangers.
- ➢ May I be happy and loved.
- ➢ May I be well in mind and body.
- ➢ May I be peaceful and at ease.

For a special person:

- ➢ May you be filled with loving-kindness.
- ➢ May you be safe from all dangers.
- ➢ May you be happy and loved.
- ➢ May you be well in mind and body.
- ➢ May you be peaceful and at ease.

For a neutral person:

- ➢ May you be filled with loving-kindness.
- ➢ May you be safe from all dangers.
- ➢ May you be happy and loved.
- ➢ May you be well in mind and body.
- ➢ May you be peaceful and at ease.

For a difficult person:

- ➢ May you be filled with loving-kindness.
- ➢ May you be safe from all dangers.
- ➢ May you be happy and loved.
- ➢ May you be well in mind and body.
- ➢ May you be peaceful and at ease.

For all beings:

- ➢ May all beings be filled with loving-kindness.
- ➢ May all beings be safe from all dangers.

> ➤ May all beings be happy and loved.
> ➤ May all beings be well in mind and body.
> ➤ May all beings be peaceful and at ease.

Loving-Kindness Meditation is a very effective way to feel that loving, caring feeling toward yourself and others, even those difficult people in your life. If at first you find that you aren't responding in a caring, loving way, give yourself more time to practice *metta*. This is a new way of thinking and feeling. The results don't happen instantly or in some instances quickly.

Continue to practice this meditation, giving yourself permission to feel in a loving way. Sometimes that's all it takes. It will be very worth the effort to continue to practice on a regular basis. You'll soon find your heart welling up with the feelings of love and compassion for yourself and all the others that are a part of your meditation.

SECTION 6

EMOTIONAL FREEDOM
TECHNIQUE (EFT)

EFT Script: Tapping for Anxiety
EFT Script: Tapping for Overwhelm
EFT Script: Tapping for Stress Relief
EFT Script: Tapping for Restful Sleep

EMOTIONAL FREEDOM TECHNIQUE (EFT)

ALL ABOUT EFT

THIS SECTION IS on a relatively new healing tool for many of us, the Emotional Freedom Technique (EFT). Even though its origin lies in ancient Chinese medicine, and it has been used in Eastern cultures for over five thousand years, it is just now becoming widely recognized in the Western world. For short, it is often called EFT or tapping. Throughout this book, I'll refer to the Emotional Freedom Technique simply as tapping.

Tapping is a gentle, easy-to-learn, noninvasive, and very effective treatment for an impressive list of conditions, both physical and psychological, that combines the ancient practice of acupuncture and modern psychological talk therapy. Gary Craig is credited as the founder of EFT and has many videos that are helpful for beginners, which an Internet search will confirm.

Tapping is often likened to acupuncture except without the needles. No needles is definitely one of its biggest pluses! In Chinese acupuncture, needles are inserted in special energy meridians or energy pathways throughout the body to remove any energy blockages. The removal of the energy blockages then allows the energy, called chi, to flow through the cells of the body unobstructed.

According to Chinese acupuncturists, removing the energy blockages also removes negative emotions. This reestablishes the balance of the chi's energy flow throughout the body, restoring well-being and health, both physical and emotional, to the person.

Unlike acupuncture, in tapping the tips of the fingers are used instead of needles to stimulate the same acupressure points throughout the body. Two or three fingers of either hand or both hands are used to tap on the predetermined acupressure points, mainly on the head and upper torso, thus the name "tapping."

Along with stimulating the acupressure points on the body with the fingertip, verbal statements are made identifying the specific problem being worked on. This combination of physically tapping on the body's meridian points and the mental/verbal saying of the problem is credited with the high success rate of tapping.

Tapping has been found to be very effective in treating a variety of physical and emotional conditions, including:

- Decreasing or eliminating phobias and fears
- Lessening anxiety and compulsive thinking
- Decreasing or eliminating physical pain
- Reducing depression and anxiety
- Addressing completion of positive goals
- Removing negative emotions associated with trauma
- Lessening the negative emotions of PTSD
- Addressing addiction
- Clearing stress from past trauma
- Weight loss
- Increasing self-confidence
- Eliminating or decreasing the fear of public speaking
- Reducing or eliminating test anxiety

A Brief History of Tapping

In 1980, Roger Callahan, a psychologist, was working with a patient who had an extreme phobia of water. Mary's life was dominated by her fear of water. She became fearful when it rained. She wouldn't take her children to the beach or pool for fear of being near the water. She frequently had nightmares about water. She couldn't stand to watch any scenes on television that were in or near water.

In addition to her fear of water, she felt intense abdominal pains. During one of her sessions with Dr. Callahan, he convinced her to sit outside with him by his pool. She immediately felt the intense pain in her stomach but agreed. While she was able to control her symptoms, the phobia never was totally resolved.

As they talked outside by the pool, Dr. Callahan remembered that in research he was studying he had read that there was a specific acupuncture point under the eye on the cheekbone related to the stomach meridian. He had an inspiration and told Mary to start tapping on her cheekbone under the eye as they sat outside by the pool hoping it would help ease her stomach pain.

The results were short of miraculous! Mary's stomach pains were gone immediately. She was so happy that she went to the edge of the pool and started splashing around in the water. Her phobia was gone too. After so many years of this crippling phobia, she was free.

Through much trial and error, Gary Craig, who trained under Dr. Callahan, worked on perfecting the process that today is known as EFT tapping. He developed the basic sequence and found that the order of the tapping sequence was not crucial. People responded to tapping easily and quickly regardless of the order of the tapping points. He did suggest the tapping sequence that we'll use in this book.

THE SCIENCE OF EFT

The science is finally catching up to what Chinese acupuncturists knew centuries ago and used successfully to treat illness. Recently, studies at Harvard Medical School have found that by stimulating the acupressure points or meridians on the body, as in tapping, the activity of the amygdala is greatly reduced.

This is important because as explained earlier, the amygdala is that small, pea-sized gland in your brain that is responsible for the fight-or-flight response in the body. The amygdala is the alarm system of the body. Originally, it was meant to warn you that the tiger in front of you was about to make you his lunch! You then had to either fight or take flight to get away, hence the name fight-or-flight.

During a fight-or-flight response alarm, the hormones cortisol and adrenaline are released, causing the following changes in the body:

- An increase in your heart rate and blood pressure to increase blood circulation
- More blood is sent to your arms and legs to aid in running or fighting
- Your breathing becomes faster to get more oxygen throughout the body
- Digestion and healing stop as the body has more pressing issues at hand
- The pupils dilate allowing you to see the danger better

All these changes result in your body being in the fight-or-flight mode in order to survive the danger. For more details on the fight-or-flight response, see Part One.

However, since we don't normally face bears or tigers in our daily life anymore, the amygdala now responds to any emotional or stressful moment in the same way it would to the bear or the tiger. It sends messages to different parts of the body, including the adrenal glands to release the hormones cortisol and adrenaline. These hormones are responsible for preparing the body to fight or take flight even though no real physical danger exists.

Cortisol, produced in normal amounts, is actually necessary for the body to function normally. It is essential to get us out of bed in the morning. It helps the immune system protect the body from any viral or bacterial invaders that mean to do us harm. It is only when the body goes into sustained fight-or-flight mode for long periods of time and too much cortisol is produced that the body experiences the ill effects.

In 2012 the American Psychological Association reported that 22 percent of Americans live with high levels of stress for a great part of their lives. Studies, such as the Harvard Medical School study, have found that tapping on the same meridians used during a tapping sequence greatly calms the amygdala and reduces the amount of stress hormones, including cortisol, that are released throughout the body.

The importance of this is that by reducing the activity of the amygdala in the body, it goes into the fight-or-flight response less often. This allows the trillions of cells in the body to go about doing what they do best to keep us healthy and happy in a stress-free environment. This is what homeostasis is all about.

A significant study was conducted by Dawson Church, an expert in EFT and energy medicine, to determine the effects one hour of tapping would have on the levels of cortisol in the body of eighty-three participants. One group received tapping with the spoken statements for the length of the study. For comparison, he had another part of the group receive just talk therapy with no tapping. The rest of the participants received no treatment of any kind. He measured the levels of cortisol in all the participants before and after the session.

The results were impressive! The average cortisol reduction in the group receiving the hour-long tapping session with the spoken statements was 24 percent. Some even showed a reduction as high as 50 percent.

In comparison, the participants who received only talk therapy or who received no treatment at all did not experience any significant change in their cortisol level. In other words, they left the session still as stressed as when they began. However, the tapping group members reduced their cortisol levels and left feeling much more relaxed.

As mentioned earlier, tapping is a pretty straightforward and easy technique to learn. A few suggestions will help you get closer to consistent results throughout your practice. While none of these is set in stone, as you begin your practice, follow these suggestions until you become more comfortable, and then you can make modifications.

As mentioned earlier, if you decide to study EFT in more detail, numerous sites online offer scripts as well as videos on this practice. There are many research studies available online. I've placed information on the Research page that will help you find many of the sites.

Here are some suggestions as you begin your practice of EFT.

It's All in the Fingertips

When practicing EFT, tap with your fingertips on the specific acupressure points on the body. There are numerous acupressure points in your fingertips. As you use the tips of your fingers, you are stimulating these acupressure points as well as the energy meridians on the body.

It's best to accustom yourself to using the fingertips instead of the soft pad on the underside of the fingers. In this way, you are tapping on and stimulating all the available points. One cautionary note: if you have long fingernails, which could hurt as you tap, then by all means, use the pads of the fingers.

Traditional EFT suggests that you tap with two fingers. However, many EFT practitioners recommend that you tap with three or four fingers. In this way, you are able to have more fingertip contact with the acupressure point on the body, ensuring that you are stimulating all the pressure points. Gently relax your fingers in a curved fashion so that all fingertips are in contact with the tapping point. Again, experiment with this to find the number of fingers that feels best.

As you begin your EFT practice, use the fingers of your dominant hand to tap on the pressure points on the body. See the picture below. Once you are comfortable with this, try to use your nondominant hand. If at first this is distracting, just focus on using the fingers of the hand that feels most comfortable.

You can also switch hands as you are tapping. Or you can go through one round of tapping with the fingers of one hand and then switch hands for the next round. You can even alternate tap. For example, you could tap on the eyebrow point with the fingers of the right hand and switch to tapping on the left side with the fingers of the left hand on the side of the eye point. You can switch fingers in this fashion throughout the whole round of tapping.

Have no concern that switching from one hand to the other will impact the results in any way. However, if you feel more comfortable using one hand instead of the other, by all means tap with the hand that feels more comfortable. As I've said so often throughout this book, this is all about what is comfortable and feels right for you. What works best for *you* is what you should try. There is no right or wrong way here.

Be Comfortable

As in all the other exercises, find a comfortable place where you won't be disturbed for the duration of the EFT exercise. Sit with a straight back, and start by taking a few deep, gentle breaths to center and calm yourself. If you are comfortable using abdominal breathing, this is a good way to help calm your mind and relax your body before even beginning the tapping sequence. Stay here until you feel you are ready to begin tapping.

If you are more comfortable standing, EFT can be done very successfully standing or walking around. Follow the breathing suggestions mentioned above until you are ready to begin tapping.

Remove Any...

Glasses because these could get in the way of tapping on the acupressure points on your face. This will become clear in the next few sections.

Watches and bracelets could interfere with tapping on the acupressure point on your wrist. I didn't include the points on the wrist in these scripts, but you could try them on your own once you are comfortable with tapping.

Also, having dangling bracelets could be a distraction. While you are tapping, you can incorporate mindfulness as well as abdominal breathing. These all add another layer of stress relief that can help quiet your thoughts, calm your mind, and relax your body. However, if adding these other practices in any way causes you to feel stressed or overwhelmed, discontinue them until a later time when you feel ready to add them.

COMFORTABLE CLOTHING

Again it's important to feel comfortable during your practice of EFT. In addition to comfort, having loose clothing allows you to practice abdominal breathing throughout the EFT exercise. This adds another layer of relaxation added to the mind and body.

TAP SOLIDLY, BUT NOT TOO HARD

As you are tapping on each acupressure point, tap hard enough to feel the tap solidly against your skin but not so hard that you actually feel pain or bruise yourself. It's also interesting to note if you are tapping very quickly or more slowly. Usually a very fast tap indicates that you are feeling very stressed or anxious. It's a good idea to slow the tapping down a bit.

Usually the recommendation is to tap about five to seven times on each acupressure point. However, if you tap a few more times, that's OK. Don't get hung up on counting the number of taps per tapping point.

Just keep in mind that if you are tapping very quickly, it might be helpful to slow it down a bit.

You can also synchronize the tapping to your breathing. Ideally, you should take one breath while tapping on each acupressure point. As an example, start the inhale while tapping on the EB point. Then on the exhale, move to the SE point. You can easily use abdominal breathing as your breathing pattern along with tapping.

As you look at the diagram of the placement of the tapping points, you'll notice that each tapping point is below the previous one. The points start at the top of your head and proceed down the face into the torso. This sequence will make it easy to memorize the correct order.

However, if you skip one point, there is no need for concern. You can either just go on to the next point without tapping on the skipped point or finish tapping on the point you are on and then double back and tap on the point you skipped. EFT is very forgiving.

TAPPING POINT PLACEMENTS AND THEIR ABBREVIATIONS

Below is a graphic that shows the placement of the tapping points on the face, torso, and on the hand. Nick Ortner, *New York Times* bestselling author of *The Tapping Solution: A Revolutionary System for Stress-Free Living*, generously provided the graphic. He is also the creator and producer of the documentary film *The Tapping Solution*. The website is included in the resource section at the end of the book.

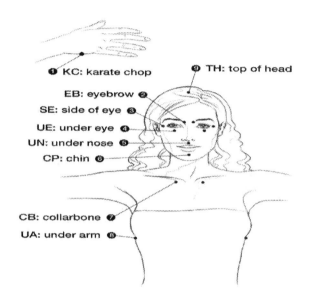

1. Top of the head (TH)
   When tapping, begin or finish the sequence by tapping with the fingertips of one hand on the top of the head. You can tap straight up and down, or you can tap in a circular motion on the top of the head. Later on, when you are more comfortable, you can try tapping with both hands.

2. Eyebrow point (EB)
   Tap where the eyebrow begins right next to the nose and over the rest of the eyebrow.

3. Side of the eye (SE)
   Tap on the side of the eye. You can tap on the bone and on the small hollow spot.

4. Under the eye (UE)
   Tap under the eye directly on the bone.

5. Under the nose (UN)
   Tap directly under the nose.

6. Chin (CH)
   Tap between the lower lip and the point of the chin—in that little hollow spot in the middle.

7. Collarbone (CB)
   Tap on the space right under the collarbone. On the graphic, it is easy to see where to tap.

8. Underarm (UA)
   Tap in the underarm area about four inches below the armpit.

This is one round of tapping. Once you have tapped in the underarm area, then you tap at the top of the head again to begin the next round.

Here is a list of the names of the tapping points and their abbreviations:

Karate chop point: KC

Top of head: TH
Eyebrow point: EB
Side of the eye: SE
Under the eye: UE
Under the nose: UN
The chin: CH
Collarbone: CB
Underarm: UA
The Tapping Script

Now that we know where the acupressure points are located on the body, you are ready to begin tapping. However, before you begin, decide on which issue you will tap. The issue can be a physical one, such as a recent diagnosis, pain somewhere in your body, or a condition you already have.

It can also be about emotional distress, such as anxiety you are feeling, a fear that you would like to eliminate, difficulty sleeping, or a feeling of being overwhelmed. Since this book is primarily about practices to quiet your thoughts in order to calm your mind and relax your body, this will be our focus here.

Many practitioners recommend that when you begin your practice of EFT, you choose an issue that is less intense. This allows you time to become familiar with the routine without the added stress of an intense issue. Once you've gained some confidence with the statements and the routine, then you can begin to tap on the more persistent and intense issues

Before starting to tap, identify the problem being addressed, and rate it on a scale of one to ten with one being "not really feeling all that anxious." At the other end of the scale, the ten is "I'm feeling so anxious that my heart is racing, I'm shaking, and my hands are sweating." Write the number down or remember it because this will be your guide as you tap to see if the tapping is reducing the anxiety and calming your mind. Say all the phrases aloud.

You always begin tapping on the karate chop point while saying the set-up statement. The abbreviation in the script is KC.

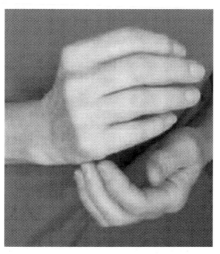

Karate chop point

The set-up statement has two purposes. The first part of the set-up statement identifies the issue about which you are tapping. Your words will acknowledge and give a voice to what you are feeling whether it is overwhelm, anxious thoughts, or any other feeling that is stressful to you. There is something powerful about hearing yourself state the exact reason for your stress or anxiety aloud.

Nick Ortner, New York Times bestselling author of *The Tapping Solution: A Revolutionary System for Stress-free Living*, uses the term "truth tapping." You are being honest with yourself as you recognize and state, as true, the issue that is causing you the stress. You can't change something that is causing you stress without first recognizing that it is the reason for the stress.

In the second part of the set-up statement, you affirm that you accept yourself even though you have this problem. You are accepting that even though you have this issue, you are still worthy of love, compassion, and kindness toward yourself. This is such an important affirmation for you to make.

Repeat the set-up statement three times aloud while tapping on the karate chop point.

Here are some examples of the first part of the set-up statements:

> Even though I have all these anxious feelings… (anxiety)
> Even though I have so much to do today… (overwhelm)
> Even though I can't seem to quiet my thoughts… (excessive thinking)

Even though I am so afraid of (fill in the rest)…
(fear of something in particular)
Even though I can't seem to fall asleep…
(sleeplessness)

You may also choose to use details that are more specific in your set-up statements that may actually help you relieve stress more quickly. Specific details tend to narrow down the focus during tapping. This, in turn, brings results more quickly and easily. Here are some examples:

Even though I have all this anxiety about my interview tomorrow morning…
Even though I have all these swirling thoughts about my physics exam…
Even though I have such restless sleep that keeps me awake half the night…
Even though I have so many things to get done tomorrow…

Now you'll finish the first part of the set-up statement as seen above with one of the following:

I deeply and completely love and accept myself.
I love and accept myself.
I accept myself and how I feel.
I love myself and accept how I feel.

The complete set-up statement could be "Even though I'm feeling so anxious, I deeply and completely love and accept myself." You are loving and accepting yourself even though you have this anxiety and are tapping to try to relieve it.

If you are uncomfortable saying, "I deeply and completely love and accept myself," use any of the other endings with which you are more comfortable. You may want to start by simply saying, "I accept myself or I accept how I feel." At some point, it is beneficial to begin to love and accept yourself even though you do have the problem that you are trying to resolve with tapping. Remember that you are still deserving of love, compassion, kindness, and acceptance in spite of this issue.

After you have said the set-up statement three times while tapping on the karate-chop point, you are ready to start using the reminder phrase as you tap on the acupressure points on the face and torso.

The reminder statement is just that: a statement that reminds you of the issue you are working on. It is generally a short phrase that keeps the issue you are working on fresh in your mind. It can be similar to any of the following depending on the reason for tapping:

This anxiety…
All these swirling thoughts…
Such restless sleep…
All this fear…
So many things to do…

Let's start by going through one round of tapping on anxiety as an example. In the set-up statement, I've left a blank for you to fill in the specific reason for the anxiety, if you choose to. If you're not sure why you're anxious, just finish the statement without adding that part.

Tap on the KC point as you repeat the set-up statement three times. Continue tapping on each of the tapping points as you repeat the reminder statement.

EFT Script: Tapping for Anxiety

Round 1: Set-up Statements

KC: Even though I feel so anxious (_____), I deeply and completely love and accept myself.
KC: Even though I feel so anxious (_____), I deeply and completely love and accept myself.
KC: Even though I feel so anxious (_____), I deeply and completely love and accept myself.

Reminder Statements

EB: All this anxiety
SE: All this stress in my body
UE: I feel so anxious.
UN: I feel so anxious.
CH: So much anxiety and tightness in my body
CB: All these anxious thoughts
UA: All this anxiety
TH: All these worries

These are general terms. As mentioned earlier, it's always beneficial to add more specific details about exactly what is causing you the stress. For example, in the set-up statement you could say, "Even though I feel so anxious about my work meeting tomorrow, I deeply and completely love and accept myself." For the reminder statement, you could say, "So much anxiety about the meeting tomorrow."

After this first round, take a few minutes to tune into your body to assess on a scale of one to ten if the level of your anxiety has gone down any or if it is still the same. If it's still the same number as you started out with, you may want to do a few more rounds using the same script above. Start the next round tapping on the EB. Since you are feeling the same about your issue, there is no need to say the set-up statement again.

If you are feeling some relief and your number has gone down a little but you are still feeling some anxiety, then you'll want to do the next few rounds using a slightly modified set-up statement.

Round 2: *Modified* Set-up Statements

> KC: Even though I *still* feel so anxious (_____),
> I deeply and completely accept myself.
> KC: Even though I *still* have all this anxiety (_____), I deeply and completely accept myself.

KC: Even though I *still* feel so anxious (_____),
I deeply and completely accept myself.

Reminder Statements

EB: So much anxiety
SE: All this anxiety that I'm still feeling
UE: I still feel so anxious that I can't relax.
UN: I feel so anxious.
CH: So much anxiety and tightness in my body
CB: All these anxious thoughts
UA: All this anxiety
TH: All these worries

At this point, again assess where your anxiety level is on the scale of one to ten. See if the number has gone down from where it was on the last round. If it has gone down, then do a few more rounds using the script above with the modified set-up statement.

If your number just isn't budging, don't get discouraged. You may want to go to the first script and do three to four rounds without any assessing. It may help if you add some other specifics about the issue you are tapping on and your feelings. This will surely get that stubborn number to budge! Once the number moves downward, then go to Round 2 with the modified set-up statement and do three to four more rounds.

If you are feeling discouraged or frustrated because your number isn't budging, stop for the time being, and relax by doing something else. However, try the rounds again later. Maybe change the words to suit your particular situation more precisely. Don't become so discouraged that you give up. This takes time and dedication. The results will be well worth the effort.

Once you are comfortable with the scripts provided here, feel free to add your own statements. The scripts provided here are more general, but you can get very specific—as specific as you want. As I've said so many times before, this is all about *you*. Your situations, fears, and anxious thoughts are unique to you, and they are producing the stressful feelings felt in your mind and body.

It's perfectly fine to create your own set-up and reminder statements that state your issue more specifically. This zeros in on your emotional feeling and its cause. When you tap, you want to address the specific stressor that is causing *you* all the anxiety. This tends to make tapping even more effective.

An Internet search will show you many variations to EFT. One tapping practitioner that I find particularly effective is Brad Yates. He often uses humor in the tapping scripts that always adds that light touch to what could be a "heavy" moment. His choice of phrases always seems to address the issues right on target!

The scripts I've provided are the simple ones that you can use as an introduction to tapping. It's good to try the different variations to find one that better suits your style. Many add a positive empowering round at the end of the tapping session, while others use the "choices statements." All of these are worth trying out and can be found by doing an Internet search using EFT tapping in the search box.

Follow the guidelines given above for the EFT script for anxiety.

EFT Script: Tapping for Overwhelm

Round 1: Set-up Statements

KC: Even though I feel so overwhelmed, I deeply and completely love and accept myself.
KC: Even though I feel so overwhelmed, I deeply and completely love and accept myself.
KC: Even though I feel so overwhelmed and exhausted, I accept myself and how I feel.

Reminder Statements

EB: I feel so overwhelmed.
SE: Feeling so overwhelmed is exhausting.
UE: I want it to just go away.
UN: I have so much to do.
CH: All these thoughts about what I have to do.
CB: I don't know where to begin.
UA: And that makes me feel overwhelmed.

TH: Feeling overwhelmed makes me so anxious.

ROUND 2: *MODIFIED* SET-UP STATEMENTS

KC: Even though I *still* feel so overwhelmed and anxious, I deeply love and accept myself.
KC: Even though I *still* feel so overwhelmed, I deeply love and accept myself.
KC: Even though I *still* feel so overwhelmed and exhausted, I accept how I feel.

REMINDER STATEMENTS

EB: I feel so overwhelmed.
SE: Feeling so overwhelmed is exhausting.
UE: I want it to just go away.
UN: I have so much to do.
CH: All these thoughts about what I have to do.
CB: I don't know where to begin.
UA: And that makes me feel so overwhelmed.
TH: Feeling overwhelmed makes me anxious.

EFT Script: Tapping for Stress Relief

Round 1: Set-up Statements

KC: Even though I feel so stressed (_____),
I deeply love and accept myself.
KC: Even though I feel so stressed (_____),
I deeply love and accept myself.
KC: Even though I feel so stressed and
exhausted (_____), I deeply love and accept
myself.

Reminder Statements

EB: this stress
SE: feeling so stressed
UE: this stress in my shoulders
UN: so much stress in my body
CH: feeling so stressed out and tired
CB: this stress about (_____)
UA: all this anxiety and stress
TH: This stress feels like a load on my shoulders.

Round 2: *Modified* Set-up Statements

KC: Even though I *still* feel so stressed (_____),
I deeply love and accept myself.

KC: Even though I *still* feel so stressed (_____), I deeply love and accept myself.

KC: Even though I *still* feel so stressed and exhausted, I deeply love and accept myself.

REMINDER STATEMENTS

EB: this stress
SE: feeling so stressed
UE: this stress in my shoulders
UN: so much stress
CH: feeling so stressed out and tired
CB: this stress about (_____)
UA: all this anxiety and stress
TH: This stress feels like a load on my shoulders.

EFT SCRIPT: TAPPING FOR RESTFUL SLEEP

ROUND 1 : SET-UP STATEMENTS

KC: Even though I can't fall asleep, I deeply love and accept myself.

KC: Even though I can't fall asleep, I deeply love and accept myself.

KC: Even though I can't fall asleep, I deeply love and accept myself.

REMINDER STATEMENTS

EB: I can't fall asleep.
SE: I feel so anxious.
UE: I can't turn off my thoughts.
UN: I'm so worried.
CH: I'm stressed out.
UA: I feel so tense.
TH: I can't sleep.

ROUND 2: *MODIFIED* SET-UP STATEMENTS

KC: Even though I *still* can't sleep, I deeply love and accept myself.
KC: Even though I *still* can't sleep, I deeply love and accept myself.
KC: Even though I *still* can't sleep, I deeply love and accept myself.

REMINDER STATEMENTS

EB: I can't fall asleep.
SE: I'm so anxious.
UE: I can't turn my thoughts off.
UN: I'm so worried.
CH: I'm so stressed.
UA: I feel so tense.
TH: I can't sleep.

The scripts that provide empowering statements do so after several rounds of tapping using the statements as in the examples given here. The empowering statements are added in the last round while tapping through all the points without using any set-up statement. Using the EFT Script, Tapping for Anxiety as an example, the last round using empowering statements would finish that session. You can also add empowering statements at the end of the other tapping scripts using appropriate phrases.

Here is an example of the last round using empowering reminder phrases.

EMPOWERING REMINDER STATEMENTS

EB: Letting this anxiety go.
SE: Letting all the stress go now.
UE: Feeling calm and peaceful
UN: Releasing all the stress from my body
CH: Releasing all this anxiety
CB: Feeling peaceful
UA: Breathing helps release this anxiety.
TH: Feeling so calm and peaceful now.

I hope that you will give tapping a try. It is a simple and very effective tool to help quiet your thoughts, calm your mind, reduce your anxiety, and relax your body. You don't need to have a prepared script. Use the words and statements that address your concern and you'll find that tapping can be a big help in quieting

PART THREE

INTEGRATING THE PRACTICES

Section 1: Daily Integration of the Practices

Daily Integration
of the Practices

INTEGRATION OF THESE six simple practices into your daily routine is neither difficult nor time consuming to do. Most can be easily incorporated into your daily activities and done throughout the day. However, it will take some experimenting with the exercises to see which one works well for you and at what time. As I've said many times throughout this book, this is all about what works best for *you!*

Deciding which exercise will work for you is strictly up to you. I can offer suggestions, but ultimately, you will have to make the time to practice some or all of the exercises consistently. I've presented what a typical day looks like and how the practices can be integrated seamlessly into your daily activities without taking up a lot of extra time.

Once you have become comfortable with the exercises, you'll find your favorite one to start your day. Alternate nostril breathing is a great way to center yourself in the morning and align both hemispheres of your brain. The number of repetitions, again, depends on what works for you and the amount of time you can dedicate to the practice.

Perhaps if you find yourself feeling flustered and anxious, left nostril breathing may be the exercise to start your day since it activates the parasympathetic nervous system, which is known as the "rest-and-relax" system. Perhaps, you may want to start your day with a breathing exercise to center yourself followed by meditation.

As you can see in the integration suggestions, the breathing exercises, mindfulness, and gratitude are easily incorporated into your daily activities as you go through your day. Once you begin to practice these, you'll find countless other ways and times when they will dovetail seamlessly into your day, even if it is a frantic one! Or perhaps, I should say, "Especially if it is a frantic one!"

However, Meditation, Autogenic Training, and EFT require that you set aside ten to twenty minutes to complete each exercise. When you decide to set aside the time for these exercises depends on your schedule. Usually the recommendation is to meditate once in the morning and in the evening. Again, that may not work well for you, so you may decide to just do one meditation session in the morning.

Because of having to tap on the meridian points, EFT is not easily done in public. It's best to just set time aside when you are at home to do this exercise. Again, there is no minimum or maximum time that you "need" to spend tapping to feel the benefits. Allowing fifteen to twenty minutes is a good beginning. If you need more tapping time, you can always continue tapping until you feel your thoughts begin to quiet and your mind become calm.

The benefits of finding—or rather, making—the time to add these practices to your daily routine are immense. You will find that as your thoughts begin to quiet and the mind returns to peace and calm, making the time for these exercises will become a top priority for you. Sooner than you think, they will fit into your day just as effortlessly and seamlessly as other activities. The result will be that you feel calm and very capable of sailing through your day even when the waters get rough!

Here are some suggestions on how to integrate the exercises seamlessly throughout your daily activities without having to take hours out of your already busy and hectic day. The interesting result is that once you begin practicing the exercises regularly, on a daily basis throughout the day, it will take fewer and fewer repetitions to feel your thoughts quieting and your mind calming. For this reason, I haven't suggested the number of sets. That will depend on your individual situation.

Here are some specific suggestions for integrating these practices into your daily routine.

Before getting out of bed in the morning:

- Start with abdominal breathing until fully awake and ready to sit up in bed.
- Continue with abdominal breathing, and add alternate nostril breathing.
- End with left nostril breathing to settle your mind and body.
- Once relaxed, go right into meditation, or do an EFT tapping sequence.

Starting your morning routine:

There are many opportunities during your morning routine to practice mindfulness, gratitude, and even abdominal breathing:

- While brushing your teeth
- While deciding which clothes to wear
- While getting dressed
- While brushing/fixing your hair
- While putting on your makeup
- While eating breakfast
- While cleaning up the breakfast dishes

DURING THE COMMUTE TO WORK:

- At stoplights, practice abdominal breathing by taking a few deep, gentle, slow breaths.
- Practice mindfulness as you remain in the present moment on the commute.
- Practice gratitude for your job, the easy ride, the beautiful scenery, and so on.
- Bless cars, trucks, drivers, and anything else along your commute route.

WHILE AT WORK:

- At any time you can stop and take five deep, gentle, slow, abdominal breaths.
- While doing various activities at work, you can practice mindfulness.
- At your desk, you can practice a shortened version of loving-kindness meditation directed at a coworker. You can say several times, "May you be happy and at peace."
- While at the computer, you can sit up straight and do abdominal breathing.
- Practice mindfulness during those long meetings by being present.
- Practice gratitude throughout your day as the opportunity arises.
- Remember all those moments of gratitude to add to your gratitude journal.

ON THE WAY HOME AFTER WORK:

- Practice gratitude for a productive, positive day filled with desired accomplishments.
- At stoplights, practice abdominal breathing by taking a few deep, gentle, slow breaths.
- Be aware of what is happening on the drive home by practicing mindfulness.
- Again, bless cars, trucks, drivers, and anything else along your commute route.

ONCE HOME AT THE END OF THE DAY:

- Feel the deep gratitude of being home after a long day at work.
- Be thankful for everything that happened throughout the workday.
- Practice mindfulness while preparing the evening meal.
- Listen to the rest of the family tell about their day with mindfulness and gratitude.
- While watching TV practice abdominal breathing.
- When the house is quiet, practice loving-kindness meditation.
- This is a good time also to review your day and add entries to the gratitude journal.

Before bedtime:

- During the end-of-the-day routine, practice mindfulness.
- End your day sitting in bed practicing left nostril breathing.
- Add an EFT tapping sequence to release all the stress of the day.
- Just before going to sleep, practice autogenic relaxation for that deep relaxation.
- Loving-kindness meditation will add another layer of calmness to your sleep.
- As you fall asleep, calm your mind and body with abdominal breaths.

As you can see, there are innumerable opportunities to practice these exercises without having to take up a lot of time throughout your day. While you are doing one thing, there is always the opportunity to practice mindfulness, gratitude or breathwork. It's just a matter of practicing awareness throughout your day, deciding which of the exercises fits in with the activity of the moment and starting the habit of doing the exercise. It's really that simple!

Of course, you'll need to consciously decide that this is something you want to do. It won't happen all by itself. At first, you may find that you forget to practice mindfulness while brushing your teeth or preparing dinner. No worries. Maybe a little sticky note on the mirror or some other simple reminder, like a chime on your phone, will help you remember until you get into the habit.

Be patient with yourself. Remember that any of these changes take time to become habits. It's been said that it takes twenty-one days to establish any habit. Scientists are now finding that it takes closer to sixty-six days to turn a regularly practiced routine into a habit. If you are trying to add more than one of these exercises into your daily routine at once, then all the more reason to be patient and not feel discouraged when you forget.

I would like to encourage you to take the attitude that if you forget to do one of the practices, you'll use this as a reminder to be more aware next time you are doing the activity. For example, if you are folding clothes, and your intention is to do so mindfully, don't be hard on yourself if you forget. Just be more aware next time you begin folding clothes that you forgot to be mindful the last time, and use this as a gentle but loving reminder to practice mindfulness.

I suggest focusing on one exercise at a time for a week or so before adding another one. This way your first exercise habit will be partially established, and you'll be on your way to practicing it consistently on a daily basis. Even if you find that you need more than a week before you feel that the exercise habit is strong enough to add the next practice, that's fine too. This isn't a marathon; rather, slowly and steadily establish those exercises into your daily routine. Be kind to yourself, and take the necessary time to establish the habit.

I sincerely wish that you try these exercises consistently and that you begin to feel the quieting of your thoughts and the peace that a calm mind brings. I sincerely hope that you feel empowered, as you quiet your thoughts, to control your mind through the use of these exercises.

I expect that if you give yourself the necessary time, you will begin to feel how powerful it is to be able to quiet your thoughts and calm your mind when *you* decide to do so. You will begin to feel that you indeed are in control of your thoughts. Even if your thoughts seem to be running wild and out of control, you know that by doing any of these practices, you can regain control again. This is indeed a very empowering moment!

Best wishes for quiet thoughts, a calm mind, and a relaxed body!

JOURNAL PAGES

Quiet Thoughts,

Calm Mind,

The Natural Way

Notes on Breathwork

_____

_____

_____

_____

_____

_____

_____

_____

_____

_____

_____

_____

_____

_____

_____

_____

_____

_____

_____

_____

Notes on Mindfulness

_____

_____

_____

_____

_____

_____

_____

_____

_____

_____

_____

_____

_____

_____

_____

_____

_____

_____

_____

_____

_____

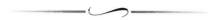

Notes on Autogenic Relaxation

Notes on EFT Tapping

RESOURCES

Breathwork

www.chopra.com
www.drweil.com
www.health.harvard.edu

Mindfulness

www.thebuddhistcentre.com
www.lionsroar.com

Gratitude

www.greatergood.berkley.edu
https://greatergood.berkeley.edu/profile/
Robert_Emmons

Autogenic Training

www.webmd.com
www.relaxationresponse.org
www.goodtherapy.org

Meditation

www.yogajournal.com
www.chopra.com
http://marc.ucla.edu/mindful-meditations

Emotional Freedom Technique

www.thetappingsolution.com
www.emofree.com
www.mercola.com
www.tapwithbrad.com

Printed in the United States
By Bookmasters